The Three
Enemies
of Your
Mental
Health

The Three
Enemies
of Your
Mental
Health

Kenza Haddock, LPCS, BCPC

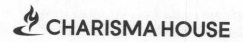

CHARISMA HOUSE

THE THREE ENEMIES OF YOUR MENTAL HEALTH
 by Kenza Haddock, LPCS, BCPC
Published by Charisma House, an imprint of Charisma Media
1150 Greenwood Blvd., Lake Mary, Florida 32746

For more resources like this, visit MyCharismaShop.com and the author's website at kenzahaddock.com.

Cataloging-in-Publication Data is on file with the Library of Congress.

International Standard Book Number: 978-1-63641-368-6
E-book ISBN: 978-1-63641-369-3

1 2024
Printed in the United States of America

Most Charisma Media products are available at special quantity discounts for bulk purchase for sales promotions, premiums, fund-raising, and educational needs. For details, call us at (407) 333-0600 or visit our website at www. charismamedia.com.

I dedicate this book to my heavenly Father.

CONTENTS

Part I: Enemy 1—the Devil

Part II: Enemy 2—the Flesh

Part III: Enemy 3—the World

Part IV: Weapons of Warfare

ACKNOWLEDGMENTS

I AM EVER SO grateful to my heavenly Father, who years ago called me into the field of counseling and assigned me to take part in His mission to set the captives free.

I'm grateful for my husband, David, who ever since we met has encouraged and supported me through every assignment the Lord has given me. I'm grateful for my children, Benjamin and Eliza, who serve as a daily reminder of the faith of a child the Lord so deeply desires for us to have.

Thank you to the Charisma team for their support in bringing this book to fruition. Special thanks to Angie Kiesling and Debbie Cole for their dedicated editing efforts on my book. Working with both of you has been a true blessing.

Thank You, Lord.

INTRODUCTION

As a clinical therapist and pastoral counselor, I've treated people with many types of mental health disorders. And as a clinical director, I have consulted on thousands of cases. Whether the issues presented during therapy sessions with my own patients or consultations with other therapists, about 95 percent of them came down to fighting the battle against what I call the three enemies of mental health.

You see, oftentimes the people I treated hadn't gotten better with their previous therapist(s). By the time I met with them they were desperate for answers. The therapies my patients received only seemed to address the symptoms that led to their diagnoses—reducing the symptoms rather than identifying the true nature of their problems. But solely treating symptoms doesn't cut the problem at its root. This is like spotting weeds in your garden, but instead of pulling the weeds from the roots, you cut off bits and pieces of them. What do you think will happen? The weeds will continue to grow, eventually invading your whole garden.

This is an apt depiction of the therapies many of my patients had received in the past. They often reported to me that they had been in and out of therapy for years without any major results, saying such things as, "I went to therapy, and things got better. But then the symptoms started happening again." A lot of my patients were in a state of hopelessness because they felt as if they were "broken," "defective," or "bound to be in therapy forever." Just like the weeds in the garden, the issues they experienced in their lives would have kept evolving until the roots of their problems were exposed. This is where the three enemies come in.

Before we jump into what your three enemies are, I want to tell you a bit about myself. It's important for you to know I'm not teaching you strictly from head knowledge. I hold a clinical degree, yes; but, more important, I have lived what I'm about to share with you and found a victory in it.

I grew up in an Islamic household, and my understanding of God was that He was mean and distant. Believing God was not loving led me to fall into the trap of each one of the three enemies to try to fix my issues. Doing so landed me in a space where I was clinically depressed and anxious for years, to the point where I contemplated suicide. (You can read more about this part of my story in my book *The Ex-Muslim's Guide to Christianity*.) Months after I gave my life to Jesus, God called me into the field of counseling. Within a few years of counseling I realized that even patients who grew up in the church, patients who considered themselves to be Christians, were falling into the traps of these three enemies. As I worked with each patient to identify their predominant mental health diagnosis and what led to it, we used strategies I will show you to overcome their mental health battles—regardless of which of the three enemies they faced.

So what are these enemies, you might ask. Throughout the next few chapters we're going to identify each one. I will describe each enemy to you, show you how we fall into its trap, and then teach you how to win the battle against the different types of mental health disorders that attack your mind.

QUESTIONS FOR REFLECTION

At the end of each chapter you will have a chance to answer questions as they relate to your life. I recommend using a notebook to record your thoughts and answers. Before diving into chapter 1, let's answer the following questions to pinpoint the key issues we'll be tackling throughout this book.

1. What do you hope to gain as a result of reading this book?

2. Do you struggle with depression and/or anxiety? If not now, have you ever struggled with these in the past?

3. If you have struggled with depression and/or anxiety, for how long?

4. What avenues have you used to try to cope with or overcome your anxiety, depression, or other mental health-related issue(s)?

PART I
ENEMY 1– THE DEVIL

Chapter 1

DEALING WITH
THE DEVIL

To defeat an enemy, you have to know its strategy. Would it surprise you to learn that the top three mental health disorders—anxiety, depression, and mood disorders—all are tied to the three main enemies we battle as human beings? Here they are:

- Satan—our **infernal** enemy

- our sinful nature, also called the flesh—our **internal** enemy

- the world, or the *unhealthy* influence of people—our **external** enemy

This unholy trinity can affect us to the point where we exhibit symptoms of severe anxiety, unrelenting depression, and/or mood disorders so extreme we feel as if we can't gain control of ourselves: we're up and down, up and down, throughout the day.

What makes the main difference between someone who overcomes his mental health torment and someone who does not (and has to come back in for therapy again and again, as if trapped in a revolving door) is the information contained in this book.

Not only will I link each of the enemies to the mental health disorders, but I will give you a step-by-step battle plan to win victory over each enemy. Each one requires a specific strategy. These steps are not only clinically proven, but they are biblically sound as well. Not only will you be able to defeat each enemy you've identified, but you will learn how to stay ten steps ahead. First Peter 5:8 warns us that we have to stay vigilant because our enemy the devil is prowling like a lion seeking whom he may devour. So we can never let down our guard. We have to remain vigilant.

The first enemy we will identify is the devil, also known as Satan. Many Bible passages refer to the devil by his characteristics. For example, Revelation 12:9 (ESV) calls him "the deceiver." He is referred to as the "adversary" (1 Pet. 5:8, NKJV) and the "angel of light" who deceives many into following his lead (2 Cor. 11:14, NKJV). We often look for this enemy to show up in ways that would make him obvious to us—for example, in a Dracula costume. In reality, as we will see in Scripture, the devil usually enters in subtle ways.

First we will uncover the devil's four-step strategy and what it often looks like in your life. Then step-by-step we will go through a battle plan to break the cycle and live in victory over this enemy. Let's begin.

The Bible says God made Adam and Eve in His image. God gave Adam and Eve authority over all His creation. He also gave them the freedom to eat from any tree, except for one: the tree of the knowledge of good and evil. God issued the following warning to them: "But you must not eat from the tree of the knowledge of good and evil, for when you eat from it you will surely die" (Gen. 2:17, NET). This leads us to Satan's four-step strategy.

1. DOUBT

This enemy entered the scene after God had issued His command. Isn't that what usually happens? We know what we're not supposed to do; then Satan comes in and makes it look so appealing. If that doesn't work, he convinces us that God is holding out on us, making the thing God didn't grant us look even more appealing. This is what happened in the Garden of Eden. The serpent, also known as Satan, convinced Eve that God didn't have her best interest at heart. Satan said to Eve: "You will not surely die....For God knows that when you eat of it your eyes will be opened, and you will be like God, knowing good and evil" (Gen. 3:4–5, ESV).

You see, as soon as Eve entertained the enemy's voice, the enemy gained a foothold to instill doubt in her mind about God's goodness. Isn't that what he does to us sometimes? We pray and seek God about buying a certain house. God answers with a no. So we begin to feel as if God is withholding from us. Or a job gets posted in the company where we work. We pray about getting it, and when we don't, we feel overlooked by God and by our boss—when in reality God didn't want us to get that job because He knew it would require us to be away from our families. We let the enemy deceive us into thinking that God is withholding something "good" from us, so we strive even harder for that "thing," whatever it may be.

Or maybe God said no about that man or woman you

have your eyes on, and you don't understand because everything about that person looks great. So you feel that God is holding back from you. What makes it even worse is that the enemy directs your attention to all your friends and family members who have found that special someone. Although God by His Holy Spirit is saying, "Don't do it," the enemy continues to whisper in your ear, "This may be your last chance to find your special someone." Thus, he leads you to pursue that person even harder and to fall into the very trap he set for you.

2. TEMPTATION

The devil is very devious. He is described in the Bible as "crafty" (Gen. 3:1, ESV). This enemy has been studying human behavior for millennia. He's been studying you your whole life. He knows your weakest points. He knows your heart yearnings. He knows exactly how to present poison to you and make it look good. This is what he did with Eve. Take a look at the following passage: "When the woman saw that the fruit of the tree was good for food and pleasing to the eye, and also desirable for gaining wisdom, she took some and ate it. She also gave some to her husband, who was with her, and he ate it" (Gen. 3:6).

How often has someone presented an idea to us—an idea that looked good on the surface—and we skipped seeking God's wisdom about it because it seemed congruent with His Word. We followed through with it, only for it not to work out. So we end up frustrated, even more doubtful about God's goodness, and feeling helpless in our circumstances.

This was the case of my patient. When she came in

for her first therapy session, she told me she was having crying spells and oppressive thoughts. My patient had lost her mother, to whom she was very close. Clinically speaking, I could have just diagnosed her with "grief" and treated that. But I dug into her past and asked questions about her relationship with God and her grief journey. My patient disclosed to me that in an attempt to find closure in her grief she had gone to someone who claimed to have access to the realm of the dead and could send and deliver messages to and from her mom.

As I worked with my patient, I discovered that she doubted God's love for her. We worked through questions such as, "Why would such a good God take away my mom?" My patient was aware that going to a medium was not of God. As we worked through steps to overcome enemy number 1 (which we will go over in a later chapter), my patient was able to deal with her grief over losing her mom, renounce her dealings with darkness, and claim her victory in Christ.

3. SHAME

Once Satan convinces us to take a step outside of God's will, often through directly disobeying God, he condemns us for falling into the very trap he set out for us. Satan's condemnation results in our feeling ashamed of what we did. I'm not talking about embarrassment here. Embarrassment is "Yikes, I shouldn't have done that"—followed by moving forward. Shame is "I am such a loser because of what I did"—followed by attempts to cover our mistakes and run from the very One who can heal us.

The latter is what happened with Adam and Eve. Take a look at what happened after they sinned.

> Then the eyes of both of them were opened, and they realized they were naked; so they sewed fig leaves together and made coverings for themselves. Then the man and his wife heard the sound of the LORD God as he was walking in the garden in the cool of the day, and they hid from the LORD God among the trees of the garden. But the LORD God called to the man, "Where are you?" He answered, "I heard you in the garden, and I was afraid because I was naked; so I hid."
>
> —GENESIS 3:7–10

4. HIDING

Hiding often comes in the form of isolation. In our shame we distance ourselves from God. This is exactly where Satan wants us.

Think about it: you and I are no match for the devil. The person he's really scared of is our Father. So if Satan can tempt us to doubt God's goodness and love toward us, fall into sin and temptation, and condemn us into shame, he knows he can get us to hide and run away from the very One we need—our heavenly Father.

The reason I began with Adam and Eve is to highlight the importance of trusting in God as the ultimate source of wisdom. Not doing so entraps us in Satan's camp. Just as with Adam and Eve, and just as we will see throughout the next few pages, the enemy's tactic is to get us to doubt God. As soon as we fall into not looking to God as the ultimate source of wisdom, we give the enemy a foothold in our lives.

In my book *Your Three Inherent Needs,* I put a great emphasis on clinging to God's goodness and sovereignty in our lives. It is often when we doubt God's sovereignty over our lives that we start looking to other means of guidance, for example, astrology, horoscopes, and other methods we will discuss in the next chapter. When we doubt God's goodness, we fall into the trap of trying to "achieve" a sense of peace and harmony through New Age practices such as feng shui and chakras, which we will also go over in the next chapter. In the meantime, please remember the four-step strategy the enemy uses in your life so you can catch it before it gets too far.

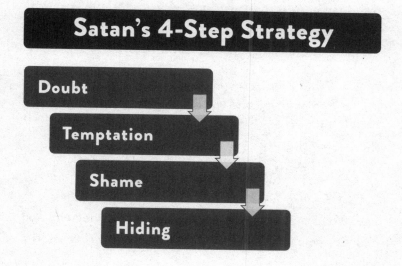

Satan's 4-Step Strategy

Doubt

Temptation

Shame

Hiding

QUESTIONS FOR REFLECTION

1. Write about a recent time in which the devil tempted you to doubt God's goodness.

The Bible says that God is faithful not to let you be tempted beyond what you can bear. When the enemy tempts you, God will provide you with a way out. Many people ask, "Well, why does God *allow* me to be tempted?" Although God Himself doesn't tempt you, He may allow the enemy to tempt you as a way to test you. Testing someone's ability to remain resilient under pressure is essential in evaluating their effectiveness.

2. Write about a time in which the enemy tempted you and you succumbed to the temptation. What happened? What were the red flags that you were headed in the wrong direction?

Red flags can often be noticed in our thought process. You spiral into negative thinking about yourself, God, and others and entertain negative thoughts such as the following:

- Negative thoughts about yourself: "I'm such a loser," "I'm so ugly," "Why would anyone ever want to be with me?"

- Negative thoughts about God: "God doesn't care about me"; "Where was God when _____?"; "If God doesn't answer my prayer, I'll need to do something about this."

- Negative thoughts about others: "Why does he/she get what he/she wants, and I don't?"; "He/she always has his/her act together while I'm struggling over here, and no one seems to care."

When we don't address the red flags, we risk going down a spiral that will be hard to come out of and end up acting in ways we will be ashamed of later on.

3. What is something you've done in your past for which you continue to condemn yourself?

Self-condemnation may give you the illusion of self-control. But it only works until you exhaust your will to restrain yourself. Self-control is a fruit of the Spirit, not a fruit of your will. If you've identified a sin, mistake, or situation in your past for which you still condemn yourself, write it down in your notebook.

4. Why do we choose to hide instead of humbling ourselves before our Father and seeking His forgiveness?

Chapter 2

THE REALM OF SATAN

YOU WOULDN'T BELIEVE how many times I've been asked such questions as, "I believe in God. What's wrong with looking at my horoscope every once in a while?" "What's the harm in wearing crystal bracelets to ward off negativity?" "What's wrong with going to a fortune teller just for fun?" or "What's wrong with trying out chakras?"

Throughout Scripture, God issues warnings against seeking any sort of guidance apart from Him. Many of the practices we will talk about may seem harmless, but they open doors that give the devil access to your life. In Colossians 2:2–8, Paul says it this way:

> My goal is that they may be encouraged in heart and united in love, so that they may have the full riches of complete understanding, in order that they may know the mystery of God, namely, Christ, in whom are hidden all the treasures of wisdom and knowledge. I tell you this so that no one may deceive you by fine-sounding arguments. For though I am absent from you in body, I am present with you in spirit and delight to see how disciplined you are and how firm your faith

in Christ is. So then, just as you received Christ Jesus as Lord, continue to live your lives in him, rooted and built up in him, strengthened in the faith as you were taught, and overflowing with thankfulness. See to it that no one takes you captive through hollow and deceptive philosophy, which depends on human tradition and the elemental spiritual forces of this world rather than on Christ.

In other words, in Jesus you find everything you need. In Jesus there's no need to search out other methods or mysteries to try to find answers. God is the author of wisdom, and as His child in Jesus you have full access to Him. Hebrews 4:14–16 says,

Therefore, since we have a great high priest who has ascended into heaven, Jesus the Son of God, let us hold firmly to the faith we profess. For we do not have a high priest who is unable to empathize with our weaknesses, but we have one who has been tempted in every way, just as we are—yet he did not sin. Let us then approach God's throne of grace with confidence, so that we may receive mercy and find grace to help us in our time of need.

So whatever you're going through that's tempting you to seek answers outside of God, just know that any answers you receive outside of Jesus are a counterfeit to the truth. The reason God issues these warnings is to protect you from deception. He wants what's best for you. That's why

He sent Jesus to save you. God also knows that seeking wisdom from any of the following practices will lead you down a dangerous path—which is exactly where the enemy wants you. Here I've listed the most common divination practices. You will find a brief description of each and why as a child of God you must not partake in it. Let's get started.

Angel Worship—putting angels in the place of God as objects of our worship. In Jesus we have access to God. We don't need to go through angels, nor do we need to rely on angels for protection. It is true that God may choose to dispatch angels to fight your battles in the spiritual realm or for other purposes. But this remains at God's discretion. Praying to angels is a form of idolatry because you would be relying on them for a sense of protection that only God can give you. And although doing so may give you the placebo effect of a false sense of security, it's not only ineffective because angels are created beings, but it opens the door to your receiving false revelation from the enemy. In Colossians 2:18, Paul's warning against false teachings includes the prohibition of angelic worship.

God is your protector. Colossians 2:9–10 tells us, "For in Christ all the fullness of the Deity lives in bodily form, and in Christ you have been brought to fullness. He is the head over every power and authority." Jesus is your Savior. He is the One who redeemed you. God alone is worthy of your worship and adoration.

Astrology (includes *astrocartography*)—the act of using the positions of stars and planets as a guide for your destiny. In the next chapter I will share real-life stories about people, including myself, who fell into this trap for years. This is a subtle trap that may begin as something fun; yet before you know it you get in the habit of looking to stars and planets to make your next move in life. Jesus is the author and finisher of your faith (Heb. 12:2, NKJV). By the Holy Spirit, He guides you through the best course for your life. God knows you will face uncertainties in this life, and that's why He encourages you to ask Him for wisdom (Jas. 1:5). When you ask Him, God promises not to turn you away and to guide you.

One of my favorite verses to lean on when I need God's guidance is the promise He gave us in Psalm 32:8: "I will instruct you and teach you in the way you should go; I will counsel you and watch over you."

Chakras—a type of energy healing that claims to connect you to the "divine"—in this case, Satan. Unfortunately, this practice is growing among therapists nationwide. Many well-meaning mental health therapists are falling right into Satan's trap by taking classes in this methodology and providing it to their patients, believing it's good for them. The Bible is very clear that Jesus is the only way to God (John 14:6). We can't access God in our own power, even if we want to. Using energy channels to try to access God's holy throne room is the enemy's plan to steer us away from truth. Sadly, so many people have fallen into this trap, seeing it as innocent and even claiming that it works. In reality, the being they're accessing is a fallen spirit pretending to be God.

Channeling—the act of calming your mind to allow your subconscious to speak to you about who you are and guide you through the best course of your life. Receiving guidance from any spirit other than the Holy Spirit is a form of divination that opens you up to Satan's realm. If you've practiced this in the past, I can assure you that the spirit guiding you was not the Holy Spirit but a fraudulent spirit of Satan's. The Bible says that Satan himself masquerades as an angel of light (2 Cor. 11:14).

Crystals—a common New Age practice that promises healing of certain emotional, spiritual, and physical ailments or protection from harm through wearing rocks of different colors and substances. The use of crystals is a form of idolatry that is detestable to God. God put His Holy Spirit in you as His child, making your body a temple of the Holy Spirit (1 Cor. 3:16). Part of surrendering to God means trusting that He will protect you from harm. God does not need help from crystals, nor does He condone the use of them as an additional form of protection. If you are wearing a crystal bracelet or have crystals by your window or in a pouch somewhere, it's no coincidence you are reading this. God is trying to reach you and encourage you that He is with you and that you don't need any other form of protection than Him. Throw that stuff away.

Dream Catchers—objects designed to manipulate the spirit realm by "trapping" bad or evil dreams through feathers on a hoop. The problem with this method is that you are placing your faith in an object instead of God, which is a form of idolatry. You may not be bowing down to the dream catcher per se, but you are putting your trust in it for protection throughout the night. The next time you need comfort from nightmares, look to your heavenly Father. Psalm 121:5–6 (NLT) says, "The LORD himself watches over you! The LORD stands beside you as your protective shade. The sun will not harm you by day, nor the moon at night."

Familiar Spirits—fallen angels that mimic your dead family members. They attempt to give you messages from your dead relatives or act like your dead relatives, depending on the type of session you're having with a medium. This act is one of the ways Satan tries to deceive you into falling for a false source of comfort instead of relying on God for comfort. Satan loves to prey on people's emotions, and this is one of the ways he does it.

Feng Shui—an ancient practice to achieve peace and harmony by manipulating external forces around you. This practice is based on a Taoist philosophy used to determine which area of a home is positive or negative; based on this, decisions about how to arrange furniture are made. Feng shui is a popular aesthetic practice among Christian households.

In fact, many well-meaning Christians who follow this practice have gone as far as rearranging furniture, hanging mirrors, and placing certain objects in the home to bring in "good energy." The problem with using this method is you're putting your faith in a belief system that is not biblical. There's nothing wrong with organizing your home, but when your decisions are driven by the hope to attain peace, harmony, or any other value that feng shui claims to provide, your hope is in a thing and not in God. As a child of God, you find peace, love, joy, and the other fruit of the Holy Spirit only in Jesus (Gal. 5:22).

Horoscopes—seeking to know the trajectory of your life through the placement of planets and constellations associated with your birthday. Reading your daily horoscope may seem like a harmless act, but in reality doing so is a form of divination that opposes God's Word. Acts 16 tells us a story of a girl who practiced divination and how the apostle Paul dealt with her (Acts 16:16–18). God is the God of our lives, and His Word warns us against relying on anything or anyone but Him for daily direction in our lives.

Hypnosis—a therapeutic practice that leads to an altered state of consciousness. Hypnosis has been used to help people process through trauma or alter destructive behaviors that were stored in their unconscious mind. The treatment that accompanies hypnosis is like downloading a file into your mind without running it through your conscious state.

Anytime you want to engage in hypnosis, I highly recommend you go to a Christian counselor who is certified in this method. I say this for two reasons: 1) While you're in a hypnotic state, a Christian or biblical counselor is less likely to download something that is incongruent with God's Word into your mind. 2) Over the last few decades, hypnosis training conferences have included New Age methods that open you up to the influence of fallen spirits. When not used in a therapeutic context, I would advise against going to a hypnotist show for fun, as this can carry its own dangers. First Peter 5:8 exhorts us, "Be self-controlled and alert. Your enemy the devil prowls around like a roaring lion looking for someone to devour."

Mediums—people who claim to have the ability to bring you closure through accessing your dead relatives, a practice known as necromancy. So many of my patients have fallen for this trap, and while the closure provided some comfort in the short term, they gravitated toward going back to the medium instead of relying on God, who is the source of peace and comfort. Mediums have a contract with familiar spirits (the fallen angels we discussed earlier). Some mediums may even claim they are gifted by God to conduct their business, but you don't have to read far in the Bible to see that God prohibits these practices. Beware of these people. They are wolves in sheep's clothing!

Numerology—a practice based on the belief that your date of birth can dictate your behavior and temperament. Numerology may seem harmless in the beginning, but it opens the door to your receiving guidance from Satan's realm. God created you in His image (Gen. 1:26) for His plans and purposes (Eph. 2:10). Instead of wasting your time looking to "numbers," seek the One who made you for answers about His plans and purposes for your life. I promise, you won't be disappointed!

Palm Reading—a practice that claims that looking into your hand can give you an inclination of the predetermined course of your life. Again, this practice steers you to look to your hand to determine what the future may entail, instead of seeking God's hand and His direction, as He tells us to. The devil monopolizes on people's fear of the unknown and offers them a "solution" that ultimately leads them to seek his leading instead of God's.

Reiki—a practice used by counseling offices and medical spas that claims to bring spiritual healing to your body by channeling certain energies into it. The Bible is very clear that Jesus is our spiritual Healer. By dying on the cross for our sins, He restored our relationship with God, thus healing us spiritually. In Jesus you have access to your heavenly Father, who is sovereign over all illnesses, ailments, and any spiritual issue that may come your way.

Sage—the practice of burning a plant in order to ward off evil spirits. A plant has no power over the spirit realm. The only One who has power and authority over darkness is the Lord Jesus Christ.

Spirit Animals—identifying yourself with an animal or believing you need to be assigned a spirit animal to guide you through life. Plain and simple, you were made in God's image. Please don't reduce yourself to this.

Spirit Guides—a practice that teaches we are assigned spirit guides to watch over us from a young age. First Timothy 4:1 warns us about following this belief: "The Spirit clearly says that in later times some will abandon the faith and follow deceiving spirits and things taught by demons." Believing in spirit guides or following the guidance of any spirit other than the Holy Spirit is a deception from the evil one—Satan.

Tarot Cards—cards used by psychics to predict the future of their clients. This is a form of divination that is explicitly forbidden in the Bible. By using tarot cards, you're stepping outside of God's will and opening the door for Satan's grip on your life.

Yoga—a practice that attempts to unify your body with the "infinite." The most controversial practice in this list, yoga is often seen as a series of stretches or exercises to help you improve your physical health. But the word *yoga* means "union," and the mantras people often repeat during yoga exercises are congruent with attempts to resolve life's toughest questions through transcendental meditation and connection to the infinite. Are body stretches bad? No. But any time we engage in something that involves unbiblical practices, we're opening ourselves up to giving Satan access to our lives.

There are many other practices I didn't include here. Honestly, I often don't explain each one of these practices to my patients because I don't want to give the practices any power over a person's life. But the practices I included above are the ones I've been asked to clarify during therapy sessions. I wanted to give you the most biblical and practical information on them to help you understand why they must be renounced—to close the door to the kingdom of darkness and live the victorious life Christ wants you to live.

QUESTIONS FOR REFLECTION

I have yet to meet with a patient who has not engaged in at least one or two of the practices mentioned in this chapter. On average, a person engages in four to six—especially nowadays, when some of these practices are socially acceptable and even encouraged. In the next chapter I'll divulge which practices I've engaged in, and then we'll dive into how to close the door to the "legal" access the enemy gained through those practices. For now, let's figure out which accesses he's taken ahold of by your engagement.

1. Out of the list of practices, which ones have you tried?

2. What made you gravitate toward those practices?

Chapter 3

DABBLING IN THE DARK SIDE

NYTIME WE TRY to seek knowledge outside of God, we are opening the door to Satan. Throughout this chapter I will share stories of patients who fell into Satan's strategy and dabbled with the dark side. If one of these stories resonates with you, know that you can turn back to the One who loves you most and win the battle against your adversary, Satan.

CASE 1: THE MISGUIDED COUNSELOR

Take Tracy, for example, a once successful counselor who dabbled in the dark side, and it ended up wreaking havoc in her life. Tracy had a busy and popular therapy practice. Her patients loved her. To tweak her portfolio, she decided to learn new specialties, so she trained in New Age therapeutic modalities. A few weeks after she came back from her seminars, she complained of all types of physical and emotional ailments she hadn't had before. In the weeks that followed, my friend reported books flying off her shelves during sessions.

To try to stop the chaos, Tracy invited a witchdoctor to "pray" over the entire building. My office was in the same building, by the way, so I proceeded to pray over my office. I tried warning my friend about the dangers of engaging with the spiritual realm without Jesus, but she quickly switched the subject to how she visited a palm reader who got her in touch with her dead father. I told her the person she spoke to wasn't her dead father but a familiar spirit— an imposter spirit who acted like it was her father. Tracy denied that her ailments and strange occurrences had anything to do with her newfound interest in New Age practices, and despite my warnings she refused to see the dangers of engaging in New Age practices.

Every time I brought up Jesus, she answered, "I'll go to church with you sometime." I tried to explain that Jesus was more interested in a relationship than mere rituals, but she seemed uninterested. It was clear that she was more captivated by the unseen realm than by having a relationship with the One who has authority over the seen and the unseen.

Unfortunately, Tracy's flirtation with darkness turned into a full immersion. One day she informed me that she had invited a group of friends to "cleanse" the whole office using spiritual chants. She asked if I was interested in having my room cleansed. I said no. The more I warned her about the dangers of engaging with darkness, the more distant our relationship grew, to the point that we became mere acquaintances. Within a few years, my friend's emotional condition worsened, and she was no longer able to practice counseling. We lost touch.

Darkness can seem captivating because it offers "guidance" that may seem innocent in the beginning. But once your foot is in the door, so to speak, it can flip your life upside down, just as it did my friend's. If you've engaged in the dark realm at any point in your life, we will go over steps to renounce any association with it so you can continue walking with Christ, the author and finisher of your faith.

CASE 2: JESUS + IDOL

While I was completing my internship for counseling, I practiced at an in-home therapy agency, meaning I drove to the patients' homes and provided therapy there.

A few months into this process, I met Monica, a young woman who had been diagnosed with five disorders, including schizo-affective disorder, often characterized by symptoms of depression and feelings of hopelessness, worthlessness, and emptiness. Schizo-affective disorder can also include symptoms of mania, which my patient was experiencing. She would sleep for days and stay up for periods of up to seventy-two hours, which impacted her ability to work and maintain healthy relationships and eventually resulted in the loss of her children.

I counseled Monica in hopes of stabilizing her emotional condition so she could ultimately have her children back, at least part-time. I remember the first time I entered Monica's house. She had built shrines for different gods and had incense burning to "ward off negativity." As I got to know Monica and asked about her childhood history, including her beliefs about God, she quickly replied, "I believe in God, and I also use crystals that *God made* to help me sleep, ward off negative energy, and things like that." Throughout her life she had picked up bits and pieces from different belief systems to help ease her fears and mood swings.

This is a case I like to refer to as "Jesus plus idol," whatever that idol may be. You see, Monica did not identify herself as an atheist. She believed in God. She even went as far as saying she believed Jesus died on the cross. Since Monica's faith in God's love for her was on shaky ground, however, the enemy was able to sweep in and present an "additional" solution to her problems in the form of crystals and incense. This led her down a path where she sought other avenues to try to fill the space in her heart—a space that only God could truly fill.

To Monica's frustration, it didn't matter how many crystals she had or how often she burned incense; none of her methods brought her the peace she was pursuing. As she and I worked together, she shared about her frustrations with herself and, most of all, with God for "failing" her. She not only doubted God's love for her, but she was also convinced that God hated her. And because God hated her He took away her kids as a form of divine punishment.

Do you see the cycle we talked about in the first chapter playing out in Monica's life? Her doubt about God's love for her led her to pursue other avenues, which led to shame, and now she felt as far away from God as one can feel.

During our counseling sessions, I shared some of my own story with Monica. I told her how I had grown up with similar beliefs about God and that I'd had my share of trials by authority figures. But I had found peace, the very peace she was looking for, in Jesus. As Monica sobbed, I shared the gospel of Jesus Christ with her. That day she surrendered her life to Jesus. Throughout her growth journey in Christ, she renounced all dealings with astrology, crystals, and other aspects of the dark side, a process we will go over in the next chapter. A few years after giving her life to Jesus, Monica's mental health was much better, and she was reconciled with her children.

CASE 3: UNKNOWN DANGERS

Sam initially came in for pastoral counseling to process through grief from losing her sibling. A few months into her treatment, Sam's condition got better, so we moved her appointments to every other week. One day she reported that she had been plagued with nightmares and thoughts about self-harm since our last session. As we talked more about her nightmares, Sam casually mentioned that the nightmares and thoughts of hurting herself had begun after a recent visit with her cousin. She and her cousin had gone to a store that sold crystals and tarot cards, among other things. I asked Sam if she engaged in any practices. She replied, "No way!" But she had bought an "evil eye" bracelet to "ward off any cancer and protect me from evil." She was wearing the bracelet and showed it to me.

During our session I talked with Sam about the importance of placing our trust solely in Jesus for protection from evil. I shared with her that wearing an evil eye bracelet to seek protection from evil is a form of idolatry. Since I had been working with Sam on reestablishing her trust in God after the loss of her sibling, I encouraged her to seek the Lord about whether or not to continue wearing the bracelet. She said she would.

A week later, during our session, I noticed that Sam was not wearing her bracelet. When I asked her about this, she said her nightmares had worsened and her obsessive thoughts got to the point where she wondered if she needed to be admitted to an inpatient facility. In desperation she had taken the bracelet off and asked God to forgive her for relying on the bracelet instead of Him for protection. That night Sam didn't have any nightmares! But she was now plagued with anxiety about her relationship with God. During our session she seemed convinced that God had abandoned her because of what she had done.

Do you see the cycle we talked about in the last chapter playing out in Sam's life? First, Satan plagued Sam with fear and doubts about God's protection on her life. Once she believed the enemy's lie, she sought other avenues in the form of a "protection" bracelet; then she was ashamed of what she had done and asked God for forgiveness; the enemy came back and whispered lies to try to convince her that God had not forgiven what she had done—which is unbiblical, by the way.

Through therapy Sam learned to distinguish the enemy's voice, which we will go over in the next chapter. She renounced any dealings with darkness, rededicated her life to Jesus, and clung to scriptural truths about God's nature, His love, and her identity in Him. You will find a list of these truths at the end of this book. Ever since then Sam's struggle with thoughts of self-harm and repetitive nightmares has ceased.

CASE 4: THE PAID FORTUNE TELLER

This case is best told by its author—Luke.

> Once when we were going to the place of prayer, we were met by a female slave who had a spirit by which she predicted the future. She earned a great deal of money for her owners by fortune-telling.

She followed Paul and the rest of us, shouting, "These men are servants of the Most High God, who are telling you the way to be saved." She kept this up for many days. Finally Paul became so annoyed that he turned around and said to the spirit, "In the name of Jesus Christ I command you to come out of her!" At that moment the spirit left her. When her owners realized that their hope of making money was gone, they seized Paul and Silas and dragged them into the marketplace to face the authorities.

—ACTS 16:16–19

I included this story to show you that this girl was not using "God-given" gifts. There will be many moments in your life when people will claim they are using God-given gifts to steer you right into the realm of darkness. Any time you come across a situation like this, ask God to give you discernment. God's Word says, "If you need wisdom, ask our generous God, and he will give it to you. He will not rebuke you for asking" (Jas. 1:5, NLT). God's Word also encourages us with the following: "Dear friends, do not believe every spirit, but test the spirits to see whether they are from God, because many false prophets have gone out into the world. This is how you can recognize the Spirit of God: Every spirit that acknowledges that Jesus Christ has come in the flesh is from God, but every spirit that does not acknowledge Jesus is not from God" (1 John 4:1–3).

CASE 5: MY STORY

Because I was raised in an Islamic household, my perspective of God was warped. I believed God was mean and distant. In other words, I believed He was too busy to deal with my first-world problems, and if I were to go to Him with my issues, He would judge me for them. And since I had experienced a fair share of betrayals growing up, I had a hard time opening up to people. So I was isolated— which is exactly where the enemy wanted me.

In search of truth, I turned to astrology for guidance. My research in astrology took me down a dangerous rabbit hole. I looked into Chinese horoscopes and traditional horoscopes. I read books on palm reading and numerology—all in an attempt to figure out who I was and what my purpose was and to fill a void only God could fill with the Holy Spirit. In my search for the truth, I even agreed to let my friend's mom perform Reiki on me, which, as I explained in the previous chapter, is a New Age energy practice that claims to bring healing of some sort. This practice didn't work on me; if anything, it drove me into an even worse state of desperation. I experienced depressive and self-condemning thoughts, and I truly believe this was attributed to my engagement with darkness.

Years later, after I came to know the Lord, I still felt a pull toward astrology and other New Age practices. This time, though, when I looked at my horoscope for the day, I felt a check in my spirit, as if I wasn't supposed to do it. And though I knew I wasn't supposed to, I still did.

For a while I felt as if I were fighting with my sinful nature, which we will cover in later chapters. This fight literally felt like what Paul describes in Romans 7:19–25:

> For what I do is not the good I want to do; no, the
> evil I do not want to do—this I keep on doing. Now
> if I do what I do not want to do, it is no longer I

who do it, but it is sin living in me that does it. So I find this law at work: When I want to do good, evil is right there with me. For in my inner being I delight in God's law; but I see another law at work in the members of my body, waging war against the law of my mind and making me a prisoner of the law of sin at work within my members. What a wretched man I am! Who will rescue me from this body of death? Thanks be to God—through Jesus Christ our Lord!

As I continued seeking the Lord and asking Him to remove that desire from me, God led me to renounce these practices. We will go over them in the next chapter. The closer I walked with God, the less pull I felt from the dark realm. In Christ I found what I had been looking for my whole life—unconditional love and peace that surpasses understanding. This is the satisfaction I so longed for my counselor friend (case 1) to find. This is the satisfaction I pray you will find. His love for you is deep; you just have to seek Him to find it.

The fight against Satan is an ongoing battle that often starts with doubt in our minds about God's love toward us. Once we entertain this thought, it leads us down a dark rabbit hole we can only come out of by the power of the Holy Spirit.

My prayer for us is that we would be so satisfied with God and so full of the Holy Spirit that we would not turn to anything else for guidance but to the author and finisher of our faith, in the mighty name of Jesus. Amen!

QUESTIONS FOR REFLECTION

1. Of the stories we went over, which one(s) resonate(s) with you?

2. What resonated with you in that story?

3. Why do you think God doesn't want us even to flirt with one of these practices (e.g., peeking at your horoscope)?

Chapter 4

CLAIM YOUR VICTORY IN JESUS

❝ CAN I BE possessed by evil spirits if I have given my life to Jesus?"

"I was six years old when I played with a Ouija board with my friends. I've given my life to Jesus since then. Do you think that took care of my past dealings with the dark realm?"

These are two of the common questions my patients have asked me. In fact, in my history of counseling, I've never had a patient who had not engaged in at least one dealing with the dark realm, whether intentionally or unintentionally.

To these questions, I often remind my patients that although evil spirits cannot possess them when they belong to God they can still fall under oppression and be influenced by the spirit of darkness. Take Adam and Eve, for instance. They belonged to God. They were walking with God. The enemy didn't possess them. He simply whispered lies in their ears to induce doubt. Once we heed the enemy's voice, he knows he can influence our decisions to keep us from living the victorious life Jesus intended for us to live. If that's how your life feels right now, I want to encourage you to cling to what Jesus said in John 16:33: "Here on earth you will have many trials and sorrows. But take heart, because I have overcome the world" (NLT). In Jesus we can claim victory over any mood-altering spirits.

Before I go over how to claim your victory in Jesus, I want to put a great emphasis on His authority over the kingdom of darkness. I've had countless patients who were scared of stepping into their victory out of fear of retaliation from the devil. So let's put your mind at ease by walking you through the following Bible verses about who Jesus is, His authority over your life, and His ultimate authority over the kingdom of darkness.

The Bible says, "He [Jesus] canceled the record of the charges against us and took it away by nailing it to the cross. In this way, he disarmed the spiritual rulers and authorities. He shamed them publicly by his victory over them on the cross" (Col. 2:14–15, NLT).

LETTER FROM A KING

Years before I surrendered my life to Jesus, I had a dream that I received a letter in the mail from a king. I remember my walk back from the mailbox to the front door. The moment I broke the seal of the envelope, my heart sank as I discovered the dreadful news: I had been sentenced to death. But, against all odds, a glimmer of hope remained because the king had personally marked the letter with a stamp of pardon. I'll never forget the awful feeling I experienced in my dream and how the devastating news of my sentence came as a complete shock. Previously, I had no idea of the trouble I was in or that I even needed a pardon. At the time, because I was Muslim, I believed that salvation could be earned, so I didn't understand what the dream meant.

Unfortunately, this is where the devil has a lot of people. They think "I'm a good person" or "I do good things; I don't have anything to worry about." Such thoughts keep them asleep to their need to be saved and unaware that they have a Savior who shed His own blood for them.

It wasn't until years after I surrendered my life to Jesus that I realized God had been sending me dreams about what was going to happen to me spiritually in the years to come. In His infinite love, Jesus—the King of kings, who defeated the devil—pardoned me, forgave my sins, and released me from condemnation when I gave my life to Him. The same principle applies to you. When you surrender to Jesus as Lord and Savior, the King of kings cancels the legal charges against you in the courtroom of heaven.

YOUR AUTHORITY COMES FROM JESUS

By dying on the cross for your sins and mine, Jesus showed the devil who's boss. The devil has no authority over a believer who is walking with Jesus. Jesus is "far above all rule and authority, power and dominion, and every title that can be given, not only in the present age but also in the one to come. And God placed all things under his feet and appointed him to be head over everything for the church" (Eph. 1:21–22).

Many of my patients viewed spiritual warfare as a war between God and the devil, or Jesus versus the devil. In reality, the devil doesn't come anywhere close to Jesus. You see, Jesus is God; the devil is just a fallen angel. In fact,

Satan and all his demons bow down to Jesus. The Bible says if the Son sets you free, you are free indeed (John 8:36). When it comes to your freedom from any spiritual practices you engaged in in the past, your freedom is found in Christ.

Jesus offers you freedom from oppression, depression, anxiety, overwhelming thoughts, and spiritual defeat. If this is where you find yourself, Jesus says to you right now, "Come to me, all you who are weary and burdened, and I will give you rest. Take my yoke upon you and learn from me, for I am gentle and humble in heart, and you will find rest for your souls. For my yoke is easy and my burden is light" (Matt. 11:28–30).

Coming to the Lord Jesus Christ requires surrendering your life to His lordship. Again, the devil is not scared of you; he is scared of Jesus. That's why it is through Christ, and Christ alone, that you find freedom. Before I walk my patients through their past dealings with darkness, I ask them if they belong to Jesus. This question must be settled first before proceeding, for the following reason: the Bible is clear that you must belong to Jesus before you step into battle with the enemy.

> When an evil spirit leaves a person, it goes into the desert, seeking rest but finding none. Then it says, "I will return to the person I came from." So it returns and finds its former home empty, swept, and in order. Then the spirit finds seven other spirits more evil than itself, and they all enter the person and live there. And so that person is worse off than before. That will be the experience of this evil generation.
>
> —Matthew 12:43–45, nlt

Without Christ you wouldn't have the power or authority to renounce any past dealings with darkness. People have asked me if I could use my authority in Christ to walk them through the renunciation steps without having them give their lives to Jesus. My answer is always no. As you see from Matthew 12:43–45, the Bible is clear that if a person is cleansed from spiritual darkness without getting filled with Jesus, the demonic spirits who were in that person will go back to the person. They will incite other unclean spirits to take possession of that person, resulting in their feeling worse than before.

In Christ you can close the door to any past dealings with the realm of darkness using your authority as a son or daughter of the living God. In Christ you don't ever have to worry about being possessed by an evil spirit and the Holy Spirit at the same time. Again, once the Holy Spirit seals you, the evil spirits can try to influence you. But as a son or daughter of God who is indwelled by the Holy Spirit, evil spirits *cannot* possess you.

If you don't belong to Jesus and would like to give your life to Him as your Lord and Savior, or if you would like to rededicate your life to Jesus, please pray this simple prayer:

> *Dear Jesus, I confess that I am a sinner in need of a Savior. Please forgive me for my sins. Thank You for dying on the cross for me. I receive You as my Lord and Savior.*

QUESTIONS FOR REFLECTION

1. How do you truly view Jesus in comparison to the devil?

2. How do you see yourself in comparison to the devil?

Chapter 5

YOUR BATTLE PLAN
AGAINST ENEMY 1

O UR BATTLE PLAN against enemy 1 includes
four steps. The first step is breaking ties with
dark practices. In his ministry Paul urged new
believers to publicly renounce their ties to darkness. Acts
19:19–20 says:

> Many of those who believed now came and
> openly confessed what they had done. A number
> who had practiced sorcery brought their scrolls
> together and burned them publicly. When they
> calculated the value of the scrolls, the total came
> to fifty thousand drachmas. In this way the word
> of the Lord spread widely and grew in power.

This follows the admonition to "demolish arguments
and every pretension that sets itself up against the knowledge of God, and...take captive every thought to make it
obedient to Christ" (2 Cor. 10:5). To complete this initial
step, we're going to renounce your dealings with darkness.
Before we begin this process, please pray the following
prayer:

Father, Your Word tells me to come to the throne of grace boldly, that I may receive grace and mercy in my time of need (Heb. 4:16). Father, I confess that I have taken part in the realm of darkness. As I am preparing to renounce any dealings with the dark realm, I pray against any attacks or distractions of the enemy. I pray that You will render me invisible in the spirit realm that I may complete this step and close every door I have opened whether knowingly or unknowingly. I trust You, Father, and I claim Your hedge of protection over me right now. As I break off any ties with the realm of darkness, may Your Holy Spirit minister to me and lead me into the victory You have given me in Jesus. I pray this in the name above all names, the name of Jesus. Amen.

Step 1: Take a look at the following list of practices. Once you review this list, write down the practice(s) you have engaged in and the age or age range in which you engaged in them.

Dark Realm Practices

Angel cards
Angel numbers
Angel readings
Astral projections
Astrology
Buddhism
Chakras

Channeling
Crystals
Dream catchers
Earth angels
Energy healing
Feng shui
Goddesses
Hinduism
Horoscopes
Hypnosis
Islam
Mediums
Numerology
Oracle cards
Ouija board
Out-of-body experiences
Pantheism
Past-life beliefs
Pendulums
Polytheism
Psychic readings
Reiki
Sage
Spirit guides
Tarot cards
Universalism
Wicca
Yoga
Other: _____

Practice	Age Range
Example: Tarot card reading	*14–22*

Your heavenly Father is with you right now. He wants to set you free. To ensure you close every door to spiritual darkness, before you begin renouncing, ask God to remind you of any other practices you may have engaged in that you don't remember right now. Pray the following: "Father, please remind me of any other practices I have taken part in knowingly or unknowingly." Wait for the Lord to reveal them to you. Go back to the table and write down any other practices the Lord brings to mind.

When you are finished, using the table as a reference, pray the following: "Father, I confess [practice]. Please forgive me. I renounce [practice] out of my life in the name of Jesus."

Example:

> *Father, I confess going to a medium and engaging in tarot card reading when I was fourteen. I ask for Your forgiveness. I renounce this practice out of my life in the name of Jesus. Lord, I also confess to playing with a Ouija board when I was eight, and I ask for Your forgiveness. Lord, I renounce this practice out of my life in the name of Jesus.*

Once you're finished confessing, asking for forgiveness, and renouncing each dealing with the realm of darkness, pray the following:

> *Father, thank You for Your grace, mercy, and forgiveness. I ask that You close that door by Your Holy Spirit and fill every void in me in the name of Jesus. I plead the blood of Jesus over my life. Thank You, Father, for sealing me with Your Holy Spirit in Jesus' name. Amen.*

Step 2: Get rid of any objects you used to seek wisdom outside of God (e.g., the ouija board in the attic; crystals or amulets you've been wearing or have placed around your home, office, car; the astrology apps on your phone—delete them!).

Step 3: Play a worship song and praise God for the victory He has given you over the kingdom of darkness, and commit to spending time with the Lord daily. Your heavenly Father loves you more than anyone ever could. He wants to develop a relationship with you. The way I've encouraged my patients to spend time with God is exactly how I've done it in my life. Get in the habit of reading your Bible. Journal as a way of sharing your thoughts with God. Seek God's direction in the little matters and the big matters, and believe He cares about every detail of your life. Talk to God throughout the day. This helps you remain conscious of His loving presence with you. It also has the capacity to calm your anxiety, depression, and any fear you may be feeling.

Step 4: Learn to distinguish between God's voice and the enemy's. Throughout your life the devil will come at you with accusations. The Bible refers to these as "flaming arrows" (Eph. 6:16). The longer you spend time with God, the more likely you will be able to distinguish the enemy's condemning voice from God's loving voice. For example, a thought such as "I'm a mistake" is not from God. God's Word says that before the foundations of the world and out of His loving nature God chose to adopt you as His child (Eph. 1:4–5).

Please note that these are not mere "words of affirmation"; these are God's truths about you. God's Word is able to pierce through the enemy's lies (Heb. 4:12) and fill you with His truth.

THE ENEMY'S LIES VERSUS GOD'S TRUTH

Years ago I experienced severe anxiety following the birth of my son. I pleaded with the Lord to take away the anxiety. Nothing helped. The anxiety became so severe I ended up at the ER on a few occasions, thinking I was having a heart attack. If you've ever experienced a panic attack or anxiety, you know how terrible it can be. In the months that followed, as my hormones stabilized, the anxiety went away. For years after this experience I felt as if I had been robbed of the first couple of weeks of my son's life. The enemy had a field day with me. He'd whisper such things as, "Isn't God able to do anything? Why didn't He give you relief when you were pleading with Him? The God who split the sea didn't lift His finger to heal you."

Unfortunately, the enemy's attempt to send me on a rabbit trail succeeded. Knowing that my son was my first flesh-and-blood relative after cutting ties with my family of origin, and knowing the importance my son carried in my life, the enemy proceeded to whisper, "Well, there goes your bond with your son, and there's nothing you can do about it."

One day I was driving and sobbing, tormented by the enemy. In my whole experience of walking with God, I've heard His audible voice two times. That day was one of them. The Lord interrupted what I believed were my own thoughts and said, "Don't listen to your enemy."

That day I realized two things: 1) when the deceiver whispers into our minds, he tricks us into believing they're our own thoughts. How often do you say to yourself, "I'm stupid," or look in the mirror and say, "Ugh! I'm so fat"? Or "I'm such a loser"? Where do you think those thoughts originate from? You? Think again. Demons are working overtime planting seeds, hoping some of them will land on soft soil. Once those seeds take root, you start repeating the same monologue demons worked hard to plant in your mind—thus doing their work for them; 2) we have a choice whether to listen to the enemy or not. But we first have to learn to discern his voice from God's voice.

God's voice is not condemning. God may convict you,

but His conviction is specific to your behavior because the way you behaved was out of alignment with who you are in Christ. So when God convicts you, He does it to restore you. The devil, on the other hand, attacks your identity. He knows that in Christ he can't change your spiritual DNA, so he comes at you with accusations. He knows that if he persists long enough and you listen to his lies long enough, you'll start to believe them.

I've included a chart here as an example. Please note that these are not mere words of affirmation; these are God's truths about you. God's Word is able to pierce through the enemy's lies (Heb. 4:12) and fill you with His truth. Just as the enemy's lies have the capacity to take root in your heart, so can God's truth.

As you use the following table to help you learn how to distinguish between God's voice and Satan's voice, please note that it is helpful to take God's Word and personalize it by using "I" statements. Choose one or two statements that resonate with you and repeat them to yourself daily over the next couple of weeks. As you do this, you will be asserting God's truth over the enemy's lies, and in doing so you will be creating new neural connections in your brain that are based on God's truth. These new neural connections will generate new thought patterns that are in alignment with who you are in Christ.

The Enemy's Voice	God's Voice
I'm ugly.	I was made in the image of God (Gen. 1:26).

The Enemy's Voice	God's Voice
I'm not good enough.	I was chosen by God out of His love for me; that alone is enough (Eph. 1:4).
I'm so far behind where I need to be in life.	I am confident that God, who began a good work in me, will carry it to completion (Phil. 1:6).
God is too busy for my prayers.	In Jesus, I can approach God confidently (Heb. 4:16).
God is tired of my mistakes.	God's mercies are new for me every day (Lam. 3:22–23).
God is mad at me.	Nothing can separate me from the love of God that is in Christ Jesus (Rom. 8:38–39).

In the next section we will take a look at enemy 2—the flesh, otherwise known as our sinful nature. Incredibly powerful yet deceptively subtle, this enemy may be responsible for leading more Christians astray than the other two. But God has not left us defenseless. Far from it!

QUESTIONS FOR REFLECTION

1. Did you know that your enemy will whisper thoughts in your mind in the first person? Here's an example: "I am unlovable; there must be something wrong with me."

2. Which of the thoughts listed in this chapter does he whisper in your mind?

Anytime the enemy whispers a lie to you about yourself, commit to speaking the Word that directly combats it *out loud.* I tell my patients, "You may feel silly doing it the first couple of times, but after a while, when you experience how effective God's Word is against the kingdom of darkness, you'll never stop using it."

Here are a couple of examples to get you started. (Notice I'm using two scriptures to counteract each lie. There are way more than these, but this will give you an idea of how powerful the Word is.)

Lie: I'm unlovable.

God's Truth: "See what great love the Father has lavished on us, that we should be called children of God! And that is what we are!" (1 John 3:1).

"I have loved you with an everlasting love; I have drawn you with unfailing kindness" (Jer. 31:3).

Lie: There must be something wrong with me.

God's Truth: "For you created my inmost being; you knit me together in my mother's womb. I praise you because I am fearfully and wonderfully made; your works are wonderful, I know that full well. My frame was not hidden from you when I was made in the secret place, when I was woven together in the depths of the earth. Your eyes saw my unformed body; all the days ordained for me were written in your book before one of them came to be" (Ps. 139:13–16).

"Having predestinated us unto the adoption of children by Jesus Christ to himself, according to the good pleasure of his will, to the praise of the glory of his grace, wherein he hath made us *accepted in the beloved*" (Eph. 1:5–6, KJV, emphasis added).

PART II
ENEMY 2– THE FLESH

Chapter 6

WARRING WITH OUR
SINFUL NATURE

I F THE ENEMY can't convince you to put confidence in
him, he will tempt you to put too much confidence
in yourself. This leads us to enemy 2: the flesh. Also
known as our sinful nature, the flesh is the most powerful
yet unrecognized enemy in our lives. Simply put, in our
flesh we attempt to exert our own will over God's perfect
will. The flesh says, "I know what's best for me," and acts
on it. While we're free to exercise our will, if our will is
not submitted to God's sovereign authority, our decisions
will prove to be detrimental to us. As we'll see in the following examples, our flesh-led decisions can be harmful
to those around us as well and result in a state of anxiety
and torment.

The Bible is filled with accounts of men and women
chosen by God who failed to submit to His authority,
to their demise. One that stands out in particular is the
account of King Saul. Throughout this chapter I will recap
King Saul's life to show you how one decision after another
outside of God's will can entrap you into the destructive
cycle of the flesh.

Insecurity

God chose Saul out of the tribe of Benjamin, the smallest tribe at the time, to rule over the people of Israel. During those times God used prophets to relay His word, His will, and His instructions to the people He chose. When the prophet Samuel informed Saul about God choosing him to be king over His people, the Bible says, "Saul replied, 'But I'm only from the tribe of Benjamin, the smallest tribe in Israel, and my family is the least important of all the families of that tribe! Why are you talking like this to me?'" (1 Sam. 9:21, NLT).

You see, on the surface this may look like humility. But as we look at the full course of Saul's life, it becomes clear that his initial response was born out of insecurity—that he was from "the smallest tribe" and that his family was "the least important."

First Samuel 10:20–22 bears witness that even when Samuel called for the tribes of Israel to tell them who their new king would be, Saul hid. Verses 21–22 say, "But when they looked for him, he was not to be found. So they inquired further of the LORD, 'Has the man come here yet?' And the LORD said, 'Yes, he has hidden himself among the supplies.'" Again, outwardly this act may appear to be humble, but it would later prove to be the result of measuring his worthiness by how others reacted to him rather than the fact that God had already ordained, and therefore qualified, him. English minister and Bible expositor Matthew Henry, who is best known for his commentary on the whole Bible, said of this passage, "It is good to be conscious of our unworthiness and insufficiency for the services to which we are called; but men should not go into the contrary extreme, by refusing the employments to which the Lord and the church call them."[1]

At times we are tempted, like Saul, to allow our life circumstances to become an excuse as to why God can't use us. Though Saul was plagued with insecurity from the start, God gave him grace to carry out his new role. This often happens in our lives as well—for instance, when God calls us to a new job or a new place to live. God knows we may be shaken to our core, so He gives us enough grace to sustain us.

Throughout Saul's reign it's evident he never allowed God's Word or God's love for him to get into the fiber of his identity. Saul's insecurity drove him to try to prove himself worthy of the position God had already given him. And, as we will see in the next stage of this cycle, Saul's festering insecurity led him outside of God's will to the point where he began to make decisions as he saw fit.

POWER/CONTROL

Have you ever met someone who was on a power trip? This is often a sign of insecurity in which we try to overcompensate by "proving" ourselves to those around us. This is what happened with Saul. In 1 Samuel 10:8, the prophet Samuel gives explicit instructions to Saul: "Go down ahead of me to Gilgal. I will surely come down to you to sacrifice burnt offerings and fellowship offerings, but you must wait seven days until I come to you and tell you what you are to do." In response to Samuel's instruction, Saul goes to the place and waits seven days. But instead of waiting for Samuel to come, he exerts his own will and offers a sacrifice to God.

Just as he finished making the offering, Samuel arrived, and Saul went out to greet him. "What have you done?" asked Samuel. Saul replied, "When I saw that the men were scattering, and that you did not come at the set time, and that the Philistines were assembling at Micmash, I thought, 'Now the Philistines will come down against me at Gilgal, and I have not sought the LORD's favor.' So I felt compelled to offer the burnt offering." "You acted foolishly," Samuel said. "You have not kept the command the LORD your God gave you; if you had, he would have established your kingdom over Israel for all time. But now your kingdom will not endure; the LORD has sought out a man after his own heart and appointed him leader of his people, because you have not kept the LORD's command."

—1 SAMUEL 13:10–14

You see, God was trying to teach Saul the importance of waiting on Him and His directions. It is an important lifestyle habit that must become a part of our daily life for us to gain victory over our sinful nature. Instead, Saul chose to exert his will over God's sovereign will. Once rebuked by the prophet Samuel, instead of repenting to God and apologizing for disobeying Him, Saul came up with excuses to protect his ego.

On another occasion God gave explicit instructions to Saul about how to deal with a certain battle. Saul again acted as *he* saw fit and directly disobeyed God. Yet he offered sacrifices in an attempt to appease God. When the prophet Samuel confronted Saul about his actions, Saul gave a list of excuses—but this time Saul tried to cover his disobedience with the fact that he sacrificed animals to honor God. To which Samuel replied: "Does the LORD delight in burnt offerings and sacrifices as much as in obeying the voice of the LORD? To obey is better than sacrifice, and to heed is better than the fat of rams. For rebellion is like the sin of divination, and arrogance like the evil of idolatry" (1 Sam. 15:22–23).

In other words, what God wants for us most is to acknowledge that He is the God of our lives and to live like it. In reality, it doesn't matter what we do or how much we accomplish; if our hearts are not submitted to God, our accomplishments carry no value (John 15). God is the source of everything good we have (Jas. 1:17). And God alone has the power to give and to take away (Job 1:21). Saul's continuous disobedience toward God cost him his position as king and resulted in his daily torment.

INTERNAL TORMENT

After Saul disobeyed God on multiple accounts, God removed His Spirit from Saul, and Saul became tormented by an evil spirit. He found relief from the torment when David, who had God's presence with him, played the lyre for Saul. Now I am not claiming that every time you feel tormented it indicates God has removed His Spirit from you. As we discussed in the earlier section, if you belong to God, He has sealed you by His Holy Spirit (Eph. 1:13–14). If you're walking in disobedience to God's will, however, He may allow you to bear the consequences of your actions until you repent.

If Saul walked into a counseling office today, he would

be diagnosed with generalized anxiety disorder. This is a mental health disorder characterized by the symptoms Saul experienced in the latter years of his life. Throughout the following pages we will unpack this disorder and see how King Saul would have fit the profile for it today.

According to the American Psychiatric Association, generalized anxiety disorder is the most common clinical diagnosis in the world. Based on the *Diagnostic Statistical Manual*, also known as the DSM-5—the reference book mental health professionals use to diagnose mental disorders—generalized anxiety disorder is given to someone who presents with the following symptoms:

- Excessive anxiety and worry more days than not for at least six months. Though Saul's exact timeline is not indicated, he began to experience torment before David entered his service. And from the time David began to work for Saul to the time Saul made attempts to kill David, at least six months had passed.

- Uncontrollable worry. Saul experienced worry to the point that he was convinced people were going to kill him.

- Anxiety and worry that are associated with at least three anxiety-related symptoms. For Saul, the symptoms presented were irritability, restlessness, and sleep disturbance. The torment Saul experienced, as described in 1 Samuel 16:14–16, was so severe that he

hired David to play the lyre because that
gave Saul temporary relief from the torment.

Saul's anxiety was so out of control he went into panic mode. That means he no longer operated with logic. Saul's emotions drove him. When our anxiety is to the level that Saul's was, depending on our perceived threat, we either go into fight mode, where we try to eliminate our threat, or flight mode, where we try to escape from it. In Saul's case, he was in fight mode. In one instance he ordered people killed because he was convinced they were after him. In another instance Saul chased after David to try to kill him.

David responded to Saul's attacks, however, by going into flight mode. Considering the threat he was facing, David's anxiety was understandable. This shows that anxiety is not always the result of our hidden sin. Sometimes we face hardships as a result of someone else's sin. In those times, I'd like to encourage you to seek the Lord and trust that if God is allowing the hardship He will bring something good out of it.

Even through the loss of his status as king, Saul never once repented for his disobedience to God's Word or disrespect for God's commands. Unfortunately, King Saul's torment led to destructive behaviors that ultimately ended in his death.

In summary, our second enemy is our own sinful nature. The destructive cycle of the flesh begins with a state of insecurity. As we've seen in Saul's life, when insecurity remains unhealed, we try to assert our own power and control, prove our worth, and hide our flaws. Since God is the God of truth, He will sometimes allow us to reap negative consequences for our own actions to get us to repent and turn back to His will and direction for our lives. If we continue to ignore God's redirection, we become frustrated with ourselves, with God, and with those around us, and we end up feeling tormented in our own thoughts.

Throughout the following chapter we will see examples of how this cycle plays out in our lives and the lives of others. Until then, here's a snapshot reminder of what the cycle looks like:

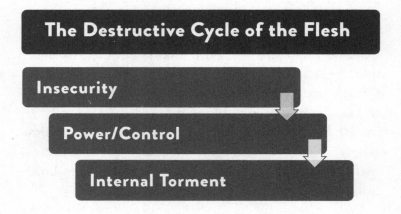

The Destructive Cycle of the Flesh

Insecurity

Power/Control

Internal Torment

QUESTIONS FOR REFLECTION

Saul's story serves as a great reminder for us to ask God to examine our hearts and keep us in check so we don't misstep toward self-glorification and self-indulgence. It's so easy to go that route. At times we may even take one misstep after another under the veil of ministry, and before we know it we're gratifying our needs to feel important and valuable—and we've gone astray from the path to which the Lord has called us.

1. What do you do when you feel that God is not acting fast enough?

2. Do you ever plead with God to do something or try to put Him on a timeline to act on something you "need" Him to act on? Why?

I've learned that regardless of how seasoned I am as a believer, the enemy will never stop trying to offer me something to ignite my sinful nature and steer me away from my Father's will. He will do the same to you. He will do it by getting you to act before you talk to God.

Here's what I've done that works: Keep your head down in obedience to God and your heart open to His correction. Keep your feet planted firmly. Do not take one step outside of His say-so. Ask Him to show you how He talks to you, and He will. Finally, I dare you to make a habit of praying

> *Search me, God, and know my heart; test me and know my anxious thoughts. See if there is any offensive way in me, and lead me in the way ever-lasting* (Ps. 139:23–24).

God is faithful. He will guide you.

Chapter 7

THE REALM OF
THE FLESH

As a therapist I've treated thousands of patients who were stuck in the cycle of the flesh. To be honest, I found it much easier to show them where Satan was to blame for their problems than to show them where they were the source of their own problems. Without fail, there comes a time during the therapy process where I must walk my patients through confronting their own destructive behaviors. I've compared this process to buying new clothes. The clothes we wear at age five will no longer fit us at age nine or ten—and so on.

The same concept applies in our spiritual walk with God. First Corinthians 13:11 says, "When I was a child, I spoke and thought and reasoned as a child. But when I grew up, I put away childish things" (NLT). As we develop our relationship with our heavenly Father, we're able to fill our minds with His thoughts about us. The closer we draw to Him, the deeper His truths sink into our hearts, filling every gap that we used to try to fill on our own. You will see this truth unveiled throughout the stories I'm going to share with you: two of my patients' stories, two biblical accounts, and my encounter with my own sinful nature. Let's get started!

CASE 1: FROM INSECURITY TO OCD

A therapist who specializes in treating individuals with OCD referred a patient to me. The therapist said the patient met all the criteria for OCD; yet she was unresponsive to all OCD treatment modalities. I initially consulted on this patient's case then decided to treat her.

"I have been to eight therapists. Do you think there's any hope for me?" Mary asked as she sobbed in my office. Mary had been plagued with obsessive thoughts about everything that could go wrong in her life. Thoughts about her husband dying in a catastrophic car accident. Thoughts about her twin boys drowning in their pool. Thoughts about dying alone. Thoughts about not being there for one of her kids if they were injured. Mary's thoughts were so overwhelming that she was unable to enjoy her kids' childhood.

As I dug into Mary's past, I discovered she had lost her mother at the age of five. Unable to deal with grief, her father buried himself in work and hired nannies to take care of Mary.

Mary was essentially left to her own feelings—a dangerous place for a child. Throughout the years she repressed her feelings to cope and survive in her environment. Her life motto became: "If I keep my feelings to myself and keep our home organized, then Dad will not be stressed out, and nothing bad will happen to him."

This method worked out for Mary until she had a set of twins. A few years into motherhood, she couldn't keep her home as organized as she "needed it to be." She experienced a series of panic attacks and anxiety attacks, which landed her in overdrive. She worked even harder and stayed up while her children and husband slept to make sure everything in her home was organized.

By the time her kids were in school, Mary had transitioned through the cycle of the flesh a few times: 1) She was *insecure* about the quality of her parenting and often referred to herself as a "terrible mom." Out of this belief, she was obsessed with organizing her children's clothes and toys and making sure that her home was in a spotless condition "for" her husband and children. 2) This gave Mary a perceived sense of *control*. When her home was not in perfect condition, she felt compelled to clean. 3) She believed this would prevent the *tormenting* thoughts she experienced over and over if she didn't clean.

As I worked with Mary further on surrendering control, she saw that the root of her issue wasn't the lack of cleanliness of her house. Instead it was the belief that through cleaning she would be able to reduce her family's stress level and keep them "safe from harm."

She discovered that she carried over this belief into her marriage and family life.

Through therapy Mary uncovered wrong beliefs she held about God. Using the steps we will go over in chapter 10, she rededicated her life to Jesus and placed her full trust in God as her heavenly Father and protector.

CASE 2: FROM TORMENT TO PANIC DISORDER

Sally was the perfect employee. In fact, her work performance landed her an executive position at her job. She initially came in to see me with a physician referral for panic disorder. During our intake assessment, Sally said she had been having panic attacks for a few months. Due to the absence of physical issues, her doctor had persuaded her to see a mental health counselor to discover if any underlying issues were causing her panic attacks.

When Sally came to see me, her professional life was thriving while her home life was in shambles. As I've disclosed to you, my therapy technique involves digging into the roots of the person's beliefs, which often start in childhood. As we dug into her past, Sally reluctantly shared that she was raised by a harsh and demanding father. She felt that anytime she met his standards he raised the bar even higher. Throughout her life, she felt that the only times he positively acknowledged her were when she received a valedictorian recognition at school and when she was promoted at work.

Sally's self-driven determination landed her promotions at work, but at home her marriage was on the brink of divorce. Sally's employer was like a father to her; in fact, her relationship with her boss reflected her relationship with her father. He was harsh, he expected her to work on the weekends, and he emailed her while she was on vacation and expected her to respond. At home, she often took out all the stress on her husband and children. She expected her children to understand what was required to excel in life.

At some point in therapy I ask my patients questions to get a sense of their understanding of God and how they see Him. Sally's understanding of God reflected her view of her earthly father. In fact, she even quoted Colossians 3:23–24 to me: "Whatever you do, work at it with all your heart, as working for the Lord, not for human masters, since you know that you will receive an inheritance from the Lord as a reward. It is the Lord Christ you are serving." I agreed with this as long as the motivation came from an overflow of God's love, not an effort to earn it. Trust me— there's a difference!

As I worked with Sally, we identified her destructive cycle as follows: Sally joined the workforce with a deficit of *insecurity*. Having a demanding boss didn't help much. She often worried about the state of her position. To *control* her worries, she worked overtime to ensure she was on good terms with her boss. When she tried to establish boundaries to have a work-life balance, she became *tormented* with anxiety about not checking emails. She was afraid that not answering her messages right away would reflect badly on her, which increased her insecurity. That led to Sally experiencing panic attacks that came out of nowhere. I was thankful that throughout our sessions together Sally followed the steps I will go over with you, overcame her anxieties, and saved her marriage.

CASE 3: THE ANXIOUS HOSTESS

Let's look at the story of Martha, a friend of Jesus. To get a better understanding of Martha's anxiety and how it threw her right into the cycle of the flesh, let's look at Luke 10:38–42.

> As Jesus and his disciples were on their way, he came to a village where a woman named Martha opened her home to him. She had a sister called Mary, who sat at the Lord's feet listening to what

he said. But Martha was distracted by all the preparations that had to be made. She came to him and asked, "Lord, don't you care that my sister has left me to do the work by myself? Tell her to help me!" "Martha, Martha," the Lord answered, "you are worried and upset about many things, but only one thing is needed. Mary has chosen what is better, and it will not be taken away from her."

Martha was the type of person who probably spent hours cleaning before she had company over. She was also the type of person who doubtless cleaned while her guests were in her home and continued cleaning long after her guests had left. Cleaning in itself is not a bad thing. Obviously, a clean environment promotes health and well-being. But when cleaning turns into something we feel we must do or else we cannot rest, then we're creeping into unhealthy, compulsive behaviors. This is where Martha was.

Martha had opened her doors and welcomed Jesus into her home. Instead of spending time with Him, though, she was distracted by everything she needed to do. She even resented her sister, who didn't share her mindset. Compulsive cleaning like this is rooted in insecurity. We feel insecure—as if a negative light will shine on us if our home is not clean enough.

To protect our image, we try to overcompensate in the areas where we feel we are lacking. In this case, we clean and clean and clean! Subconsciously that's our way of controlling our environment. And if people around us are not as compelled as we are to clean and keep everything tidy, we end up feeling tormented by the amount of work we have to do—work we put on ourselves! This was where Martha was. When she blamed her sister for not helping, Jesus reminded Martha of the importance of anchoring herself in Him. When our sense of self-worth is secured in Jesus, we will no longer be compelled to prove our worth through works. And whenever He calls us to accomplish something, we will have the assurance that He will equip us and strengthen us to do it.

CASE 4: PETER

You don't have to look far into the four Gospels to spot the insecurity Peter struggled with throughout his first years of ministry with Jesus. Peter is one of the first disciples Jesus called to follow Him. Before long, Peter became the most outspoken of the disciples and one of Jesus' closest friends.

Peter struggled with impulse control, an issue often rooted in insecurity. At times his actions may have appeared heroic, but beneath the surface they were mere attempts to overcompensate for his perceived lack for the role in which Jesus had put him. For instance, in Matthew 14:28, Peter asked Jesus to call him out of the boat. While the rest of the disciples were afraid of the storm, the Bible says when Peter heard Jesus' voice he replied, "Lord, if it's you...tell me to come to you on the water." Peter was relentlessly trying to prove his faith to Jesus.

Before we continue with this passage, I'd like to clarify that nothing is wrong with stepping out in faith. In fact, our walk with the Lord is a walk by faith (2 Cor. 5:7). Our faith, however, must rest completely in the Lord, not 90 percent in Jesus and 10 percent in our ability. As you'll see in the following passage, Peter's faith was still not completely anchored in Jesus. Matthew 14:29–31 says that when Jesus called Peter out of the boat, "Peter got down out of the boat, walked on the water and came toward Jesus. But when he saw the wind, he was afraid and, beginning to sink, cried out, 'Lord, save me!' Immediately Jesus reached out his hand and caught him. 'You of little faith,' he said, 'why did you doubt?'"

Isn't this what we often do? We step out in faith, but somehow along the way we begin to trust in our own abilities to accomplish what only God can accomplish through us. As soon as Peter realized how helpless he was in his own strength, he started to sink.

After this event, Peter continued to learn the hard way just how much his own flesh would fail him. He was the one who claimed he would never deny Jesus. "Peter declared, 'Even if I have to die with you, I will never disown you'" (Matt. 26:35). Yet when his spiritual strength was tested, Peter denied his Lord. The Bible says that after Peter denied Jesus three times, "The Lord turned and looked straight at Peter. Then Peter remembered the word the Lord had spoken to him: 'Before the rooster crows today, you will disown me three times.' And he went outside and wept bitterly" (Luke 22:61–62).

I cannot imagine the torment Peter must have felt: The torment of failure. The torment of regret. The torment of doing something he could never take back. I'm thankful Jesus doesn't leave us there. After He rose from the dead, Jesus made sure that Peter was named among the disciples who were to find out He was risen. Mark 16:7 says, "But go, tell his disciples and *Peter*, 'He [Jesus] is going ahead of you into Galilee. There you will see him, just as he told you'" (emphasis added). What a gracious Lord we serve! Jesus knew how tormented Peter must've felt about denying Him.

The Bible says, "Love covers over a multitude of sins" (1 Pet. 4:8). It's interesting that Peter is the writer of this verse. This is exactly what he experienced from Jesus. Instead of leaving him where he was emotionally, Jesus restored Peter. I believe Peter's failure was one of the best things that ever happened to him because it showed him how frail his flesh truly was. Once restored, out of the assurance of Jesus' love for him, Peter went on to become one of the greatest leaders in the New Testament.

CASE 5: MY ENCOUNTER WITH ANXIETY

For years after my husband and I were married, the enemy tormented me with fear that something bad would happen to him. Once we had children, this fear grew. I tried rationalizing this fear by telling myself it was a normal part of being a spouse or parent; but deep down I knew something was not right. Sometimes when my husband would leave our home to go to work, I feared he would get into a car accident. Or thoughts of "What if this is the last time I see him?" would plague my mind. Before I knew it, I was planning how I was going to be a widowed, single mom for the rest of my life. Other times, as I was putting my kids to bed, I would get plagued with thoughts such as "What if they don't wake up tomorrow?" "What if something bad happens to them and they stop breathing in the middle of the night?" "What if they get up in the middle of the night and fall down the stairs?" My anxiety grew to the point where I realized something needed to break through it. So I did what I knew best—I cried out to God.

The amazing thing about our heavenly Father is that He is in the business of redemption. He is in the business of setting the captives free. Referring to Jesus, Luke 4:18–19 says, "The Spirit of the Lord is on me, because he has anointed me to proclaim good news to the poor. He has sent me to proclaim freedom for the prisoners and recovery of sight for the blind, to set the oppressed free, to proclaim the year of the Lord's favor."

Jesus wants us to live in the freedom He purchased for us with His own blood. As I processed through my fears with God, He revealed that the anxiety I was feeling was rooted in my *insecurity* about His love for me. You see, I knew God loved me. But I was insecure about what my life would become if He allowed tragedy to take place. As I processed through this with the Lord, He reminded me that when He called me to follow Him He was the only One I had, literally. For months, my whole world consisted of Him and me. The Lord reminded me that when I had no one, and nothing, He was enough to provide for me. He was enough to take care of me. And He was enough to protect me.

The Bible talks about how God's perfect love casts out fear (1 John 4:18). The desire of God's heart is for us to live in His perfect love. We can know beyond a shadow of a doubt that our Father has our back, He goes before us, and He prepares the way. His goodness surrounds us. His shield protects us. When we have full assurance of God's love for us and know His grace will cover us regardless of our situation, Satan won't be able to get in and plant thoughts of fear and doubt in our minds. That door would be secure, and we are assured of God's love for us. To close the door to anxiety and fear in my life, I went through the steps I will go over with you at the end of this section. God led me to stand on a Bible verse I continue to stand on today: "I keep my eyes always on the LORD. With him at my right hand, I will not be shaken" (Ps. 16:8).

As you saw from the examples in this chapter, when we fall into the trap of self-striving and use defense mechanisms to hide our flaws, we end up feeling anxious, tormented, and fearful. Throughout the next few pages we'll look at each defense mechanism in detail and identify how each one may be reflected in our lives.

QUESTIONS FOR REFLECTION

1. Which of the stories you just read resonate with you?

2. Why?

Chapter 8

DEFENSE MECHANISMS THAT KEEP YOU TRAPPED

THE BIBLE SAYS, "The heart is deceitful above all things" (Jer. 17:9). It is quite common for us to act in a way that conceals our insecurity as a means of masking it. That's what our defense mechanisms are all about—deceiving our hearts into believing something that isn't true so we don't have to confront the reality of the very pain from which God wants to heal us. Many defense mechanisms are out there. The ones I will go over with you here are the most common defense mechanisms that keep us trapped in the cycle of the flesh. We will go over how each defense mechanism shows up in our lives, why we tend to deploy it, and what God has to say about it.

Denial is a defense mechanism we deploy to keep us from feeling overwhelmed with our emotions. When used on a short-term basis, denial can help us ease our way into the reality of a crisis that just took place—for example, the loss of a loved one—instead of having to deal with all our emotions at once. For the sake of clarity, I'm not referring to short-term denial that lasts a couple of weeks.

I'm referring to using denial as a tool to keep us from facing the reality in our lives. In my early years of counseling I worked with a lot of parents who were in denial about their children's misbehaviors. And despite what the teacher said, despite what I recommended, the parents refused to see if something was wrong with their child's behavior. The parents often said such things as, "He's just a kid!" Or "I did worse things when I was her age!" Or "That's just what kids do nowadays." It wasn't until the issue worsened—perhaps when the child was kicked out of school or had an infraction with the law—that the parents agreed to partner with me to help their children.

Why do we deny? We often deploy this defense mechanism to protect ourselves from the perceived threat we may be facing. When we encounter a problem that overwhelms us, we go into what we call fight-or-flight mode. Denial is our way of fleeing from the problem. It's our way of "burying our head in the sand" and hoping the problem will go away on its own.

The problem is that denial is not how God intended for us to deal with issues. God's Word says, "For God has not given us a spirit of fear and timidity, but of power, love, and self-discipline" (2 Tim. 1:7, NLT). We often turn to denial because we are not aware of God's loving presence with us. When we doubt whether God is truly *with us* and deny the reality that He is *for us*, we walk around believing we have to tackle all of life's problems on our own.

God just wants us to turn to Him, surrender our problems to Him (a step we will go over in chapter 10), and ask Him to guide us on how best to deal with them. God is the source of wisdom (Prov. 2:6), and He wants to guide us lovingly through the maze of life, as it says in Psalm 32:8: "I will instruct you and teach you in the way you should go; I will counsel you with my loving eye on you." We have no reason to fear that we are left to our own devices with our problems. When you seek God and ask Him for answers and guidance, be on the lookout for His answers. I've instructed many patients to do the same thing I'm asking you to do, and God has never failed them once. He won't fail you!

Repression is similar to denial but slightly different. When we deploy the defense mechanism of repression, we acknowledge the problem, but we deny its effects on us. In counseling patients, I've often seen this defense mechanism used by people raised in environments where they were to be seen and not heard. In other words, they did not learn to process their emotions properly or that it was OK to talk about their feelings and sort through them. In turn, they got in the habit of hiding their feelings and acting as if they were not bothered by what was happening around them, no matter how tragic.

Historically, people who have mastered this defense mechanism often excel in crisis environments because they know how to remain calm in the midst of chaos. They've mastered being the "shock absorber" of their environment.

The problem with repression is that it puts the weight of the world on our shoulders, a weight we were never meant to carry. In Matthew 11:28–30 Jesus says, "Come to me, all you who are weary and burdened, and I will give you rest. Take my yoke upon you and learn from me, for I am gentle and humble in heart, and you will find rest for your souls. For my yoke is easy and my burden is light."

God is not scared of your emotions. He created you with emotions. He wants you to bring your emotions to Him and let Him help you sort them out. His Word says, "Cast all your anxiety on him because he cares for you" (1 Pet. 5:7). If you grew up in an environment where your feelings were not welcome and your emotions were shut down, I am so sorry. That is not God's intention for you, and that was not His will for you. It is often when we repress our emotions that we become driven by them. But when we take our emotions to our heavenly Father (a process I will teach you later in the book) and ask Him to help us sort through them, He welcomes us with open arms and walks us through them step-by-step.

David is a good example of someone who expressed his emotions openly to God. Take a look at Psalm 13:

> How long, LORD? Will you forget me forever? How long will you hide your face from me? How long must I wrestle with my thoughts and day after day have sorrow in my heart? How long will my enemy triumph over me? Look on me and answer, LORD my God. Give light to my eyes, or I will sleep in death, and my enemy will say, "I have overcome him," and my foes will rejoice when I fall. But I trust in your unfailing love; my heart rejoices in your salvation. I will sing the LORD's praise, for he has been good to me.

God never struck David down for sharing his heart with Him. In fact, in Psalm 62:8, David exhorts us: "Trust in him at all times, you people; pour out your hearts to him, for God is our refuge."

God has never turned me away when I went to Him with emotions I didn't even understand at the time. God made us. He knows the depths of our hearts. He knows exactly how to pull out each emotion and sort through it. He will hold your hand through the whole process, and by the end of it you'll ask yourself, "Why didn't I do this before today?"

Projection is passing blame to someone else for our mistake. Adam and Eve are classic examples of what projection looks like. As we went over earlier in chapter 1, it's clear that Adam and Eve knew they'd messed up. It's also clear they tried to fix it by hiding it. When God asked Adam about the issue, Adam blamed his wife, Eve, who in turn blamed Satan for deceiving her (Gen. 3:12–13).

Why do we project? To keep ourselves from feeling the pain of our behavior. Moses experienced much projection by the very people God had called him to liberate. The Bible mentions instances when the Israelites, the people God liberated, grumbled against Moses. Numbers 14:2 says, "All the Israelites grumbled against Moses and Aaron, and the whole assembly said to them, 'If only we had died in Egypt! Or in this wilderness!'" The Israelites proceeded to accuse God of liberating them for the purpose of killing them: "Why is the LORD bringing us to this land only to let us fall by the sword? Our wives and our children will be taken as plunder. Wouldn't it be better for us to go back to Egypt?" (v. 3). For additional examples of projections the Israelites made, please see Exodus 16:3 and Numbers 21:4–6.

The problem with projection is it always points the finger at someone else for one's own problems. It rarely, however, results in humble self-reflection. The Bible says, "God opposes the proud but shows favor to the humble" (Jas. 4:6). God may allow us to blame everyone else for our behavior for a little while as He works with us on other things. But a time will come when He walks us through correcting that defect and fills us with His love, so that we no longer stand on our shaken egos but on our irrevocable identity in Christ.

Rationalization is a defense mechanism we use to justify our negative behavior. Just as with projection, we deploy this method to conceal our faults and protect our self-image. King Saul used rationalization quite often. In fact, anytime he was confronted with disobeying God, King Saul found a way to justify his disobedience.

Rationalizing our behavior puts a Band-Aid on an issue that must be dealt with. God is not in the business of pacifying negative behaviors. God is in the business of confronting what may be destructive to us to bring healing to the problem. He doesn't pacify sin. He deals with it.

Rationalization also relies heavily on intellect. The Pharisees are a great example of this. They could not see past their own head knowledge enough to acknowledge the possibility that Jesus was the Messiah. The Pharisees even went as far as rationalizing Jesus' miracles by claiming He did them by the power of the devil. To which Jesus said,

> Every kingdom divided against itself will be ruined, and every city or household divided against itself will not stand. If Satan drives out Satan, he is divided against himself. How then can his kingdom stand? And if I drive out demons by Beelzebul, by whom do your people drive them out? So then, they will be your judges. But if it is by the Spirit of God that I drive out demons, then the kingdom of God has come upon you.
> —MATTHEW 12:25–28

The Pharisees even rationalized crucifying Jesus because He didn't fit the box of rules and regulations in which they had placed themselves. They took so much pride in their self-achieved religious status quo that they failed to recognize their liberator when He came to save them. Rationalizing our bad behavior only keeps us stuck in the cycle from which God wants to free us. If you start feeling uneasy as you're reading this, maybe God is tugging at your heartstrings right now. Maybe He wants to free you from this pattern. If you believe this has been your method of coping, I encourage you to pray the following prayer:

> *Father, please search my heart and show me if there are any places in my life where I am acting in a way that is incongruent with who I am in Christ. I pray that You will bring those areas to the surface and show me how to deal with them, in the mighty name of Jesus. Amen.*

Displacement is redirecting the anger or uncomfortable emotion we have from its rightful recipient onto someone else. Take, for instance, someone who works for a harsh boss. The person feels that they can't talk back to their employer out of fear of losing their job, so they go home and take their anger out on their spouse, who then takes their anger out on their kid, who in turn kicks the dog.

Usually we deploy this defense mechanism when we believe that expressing our true emotions will result in consequences detrimental to us, such as the example of the employee losing employment. Sometimes we treat our relationship with God this way. We believe that telling

God about our hard feelings will somehow make Him mad. If this fear has crossed your mind, you are not alone! You wouldn't believe how many of my patients carried around this belief. In fact, I came across it so many times that it became a part of the homework I assigned my patients. Their homework was to spend time with God and share their feelings with Him. This type of exposure therapy was so successful in helping my patients overcome their fear that God would strike them down for sharing their anger and grief with Him. To their surprise, God did not strike them down. Some even expressed that they felt God's promptings for the first time and were filled with joy about being able to talk to Him the way they talk to me or to a friend.

God wants a Father/daughter or Father/son relationship with us, not an obligatory Sunday-visit type of relationship. He wants to be right in the midst of your feelings. And when you face a difficult situation, God wants you to go to Him and ask Him how to deal with it. I promise you He won't turn you away. I promise you He won't send you away feeling condemned. Instead God will hear you, and you will either leave the conversation feeling a sense of peace, He will give you insight about your particular situation, or over the next several days He may use a friend, your devotional, or your church's Sunday message to speak to that situation. The point is, your relationship with God is something that is developed over time. One of the most important habits to develop in your relationship with God is being transparent with Him. *Doing* is how you overcome the use of this defense mechanism—as well as the other defense mechanisms.

At the root of every defense mechanism we use is our

attempt to hide a part of ourselves God wants to heal. As we have discussed so far, we use defense mechanisms to protect ourselves from perceived threats. Our defenses are meant to be used on a short-term basis, such as in grief. For example, we may go through the initial shock or denial phase to help our brain catch up to the reality of what's going on. But when our defenses become a part of our daily life, they keep us from growing into the person God wants us to be. Before we jump into what our healing process looks like, let's talk about what our victory over the flesh looks like and how we can take hold of it as sons and daughters of God.

QUESTIONS FOR REFLECTION

Defense mechanisms are our way of covering our insecurities and protecting ourselves from pain. These mechanisms are works of the flesh and therefore don't lead to healthy long-term results.

1. Which of the defense mechanisms discussed in this chapter are you apt to use?

2. Pick two of the defense mechanisms you're prone to using the most, and in your notebook or journal write about a recent time in which you used each one.

Defense mechanism #1:

- Why did you use this mechanism in this particular situation?

- What would have been a healthy long-term way to address and resolve the problem?

Defense mechanism #2:

- Why did you use this mechanism in this particular situation?

- What would have been a healthy long-term way to address and resolve the problem?

God wants us to live in the freedom Jesus gave us (see John 8:36), and freedom requires being willing to face the perceived pain from which we're hiding. Let's be honest with ourselves—and honest with others, including God.

Chapter 9

GAINING VICTORY OVER "SELF"

W HEN WE LET our flesh rule our lives, we go back to acting out of a place of insecurity. God wants His Word to take root in us so that we are no longer driven by our old nature but by our identity as sons and daughters of our heavenly Father.

In the Book of Ephesians, the apostle Paul, inspired by the Holy Spirit, put great emphasis on making sure we know *who we are* before we are able to act according to our identity in Christ. This is because what is inside us—our core identity—drives us. When you break down Ephesians, you see that the first three chapters deal specifically with our identity. When that matter is settled, Paul moves on to our behavior in the three chapters that follow.

This method reflects the ultimate difference between the gospel of Jesus Christ and other religions. Throughout the next few pages we are going to look at a couple of passages from Ephesians as they pertain to our nature as children of God. Then we will look at how our identity sets the foundation for our call as sons and daughters of our heavenly Father. Let's dive in!

Ephesians 1:4–5 says, "For he chose us in him before the

creation of the world to be holy and blameless in his sight. In love he predestined us for adoption to sonship through Jesus Christ, in accordance with his pleasure and will." From the beginning, Paul settles the fact that we belong to God because of His loving nature. This means that God chose to adopt you as His child because He loves you. A few verses later, Paul continues to emphasize this point:

> And you also were included in Christ when you heard the message of truth, the gospel of your salvation. When you believed, you were marked in him with a seal, the promised Holy Spirit, who is a deposit guaranteeing our inheritance until the redemption of those who are God's possession— to the praise of his glory.
>
> —EPHESIANS 1:13–14

Paul wants you to understand that when you surrendered your life to Jesus and became God's child, God put His Holy Spirit in you and sealed you as His child. Now let's get to the heart of the matter!

Paul continues in Ephesians 2:1–3:

> As for you, you were dead in your transgressions and sins, in which you used to live when you followed the ways of this world and of the ruler of the kingdom of the air, the spirit who is now at work in those who are disobedient. All of us also lived among them at one time, gratifying the cravings of our flesh and following its desires and thoughts. Like the rest, we were by nature deserving of wrath.

THE GAME CHANGER "BUT GOD" VERSE

Years before I gave my life to Jesus, I had a dream that I was staring at myself dead in a morgue with a tag hanging on my toe. In the dream I heard a flatline sound that grew louder and louder until I woke up in a sweat. In that dream the Lord was notifying me of my spiritual status—dead, unable to be saved by my long list of works. Similarly, in the passage we just read, Paul reminds us that in our own flesh nature we were unable to save ourselves from God's wrath. Our nature separated us from God, and because of that we were rightfully deserving of His judgment.

Right after this, Paul says in Ephesians 2:4: "But because of his great love for us, God, who is rich in mercy...." I call this the "but God" verse—because this verse is the game changer for you, for me, and for whoever chooses to put their faith in the lordship of Jesus. This verse serves as a reminder of God's endless love for you and the mercy He extended to you in Jesus. Paul continues with verses 5–7:

> [God] made us alive with Christ even when we were dead in transgressions—it is by grace you have been saved. And God raised us up with Christ and seated us with him in the heavenly realms in Christ Jesus, in order that in the coming ages he might show the incomparable riches of his grace, expressed in his kindness to us in Christ Jesus. For it is by grace you have been saved, through faith—and this is not from yourselves, it is the gift of God—not by works, so that no one can boast. For we are God's handiwork,

created in Christ Jesus to do good works, which
God prepared in advance for us to do.

I believe Paul understood the nature of the flesh we
would be at war with constantly because of how often
he emphasized the importance of finding our identity in
Christ rather than in what we "do" for God. This is something I struggled with for years after surrendering my life
to Jesus. One day, though, God gave me an illustration to
help me understand my transition from a flesh-led life to a
Spirit-led life. I'd like to share this illustration with you in
hopes it will bring clarity to you as well.

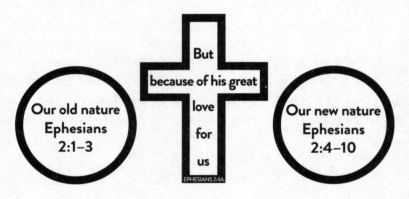

Now that our identity in Christ is set, Paul moves on to
answer the question "How do I talk to God?" In Ephesians
3:12 Paul says: "In him [Jesus] and through faith in him we
may approach God with freedom and confidence." As a
child of God, you can approach God confidently, knowing
you have His undivided attention. You never have to
worry that He will turn you away because your problems
are "first-world problems." You never have to worry that

God will condemn you for coming to Him with your mistakes. Just the opposite. God wants you to come to Him confidently about anything and everything, knowing His love has you covered. He loves you beyond measure. God's love is the foundation on which Paul continues to build his message in Ephesians 3:14–19.

> For this reason I kneel before the Father, from whom every family in heaven and on earth derives its name. I pray that out of his glorious riches he may strengthen you with power through his Spirit in your inner being, so that Christ may dwell in your hearts through faith. And I pray that you, being rooted and established in love, may have power, together with all the Lord's holy people, to grasp how wide and long and high and deep is the love of Christ, and to know this love that surpasses knowledge—that you may be filled to the measure of all the fullness of God.

Having an identity rooted in God's love is a prerequisite to letting go of all our defense mechanisms. When we experience the depth of our Father's love for us, which is at the heart of Paul's prayer, we are able to voluntarily surrender our broken hearts into His hands. Why? Because we know that is the safest, most comforting place where we could ever surrender anything.

LIVING AS GOD'S CHILDREN

Once our identity is built upon the foundation of God's love, we are ready to receive instruction on how to live as God's children. In Ephesians 4:1–2 Paul says, "I urge you to live a life worthy of the calling you have received. Be completely humble and gentle; be patient, bearing with one another in love." Humility goes completely against the nature of our flesh. In our flesh we pursue our own desires, not God's desires for our lives. In our flesh we look after our own interests, not the interests of others. Paul knows our behavior often stems from our identity. That's why he settled the matter of identity in the first three chapters of Ephesians. Once our identity is secured in God's love for us, we are ready to live in a manner worthy of the call God has on our life—in other words, a life that reflects the love of the Father.

If you have children, you can probably remember how, even when they were babies, you noticed traits that resembled either yours or their other parent's. The same concept applies to our walk with Christ. The closer we walk with God, the more we "look" like Him in the way we act, and people identify us with Him. Living a life worthy of the call we have received means that people can look at the way we live our lives and know we belong to God.

In Ephesians 4:29–32 Paul tackles flesh-driven problems that may tempt us.

> Do not let any unwholesome talk come out of your mouths, but only what is helpful for building others up according to their needs, that it may benefit those who listen. And do not grieve the Holy Spirit of God, with whom you were sealed for the day of redemption. Get rid of all bitterness, rage and anger, brawling and slander, along with every form of malice. Be kind and compassionate

to one another, forgiving each other, just as in
Christ God forgave you.

As a child of God, your circle of influence extends
beyond what you can imagine. Whether you are aware of
it or not, many people pay attention to the way you live. As
a child of God, you are an image bearer of your Father in
heaven. As God's ambassador, the apostle Paul is encouraging you to get rid of any of the flesh characteristics that
could hurt the testimony of what God has done in and
through your life.

"Unwholesome talk" was one of the toughest areas for
me to overcome, and I dare to say it's a daily, conscious
decision to make sure that nothing unwholesome comes
out of my mouth. Before Jesus, unwholesome language
was a part of my vocabulary. "That's just how I talk," I
rationalized. But as I drew close to Christ it didn't feel
good to use it anymore.

The point is, God wants to demonstrate His miraculous
power through you. How will people see God in you if you
still gossip as much as you did before you gave your life to
Jesus? How will people believe God is approachable if you
are not approachable? How will people understand grace
if you're shrewd with them? God wants to use you as His
hands and feet to those who either do not know Him or
those who hold the wrong perspective of Him. The more
you spend time with God, the more you will look like
Him in your actions.

Paul continues, "For you were once darkness, but now
you are light in the Lord. Live as children of light (for the
fruit of the light consists in all goodness, righteousness
and truth)" (Eph. 5:8–9). Many times in your life you will

feel the tension between the flesh and the spirit, as Paul described in his own life (Romans 7). During these times, know that Jesus is with you. He is interceding for you in heaven. I pray that His grace will sustain you and carry you to victory.

As God's beloved child you no longer need to let insecurity drive you because you are secure in His love. You no longer need to let your wounds of rejection drive you because you're fully accepted in Jesus. You no longer need to strive for significance because your Father in heaven calls you by name. You always have your Father's undivided attention, and you can rest assured that He cares about every detail of your life.

Finally, Paul wraps up his letter to the Ephesians with instructions to make sure we don't fall asleep in the ongoing spiritual battle.

> Put on the full armor of God, so that you can take your stand against the devil's schemes. For our struggle is not against flesh and blood, but against the rulers, against the authorities, against the powers of this dark world and against the spiritual forces of evil in the heavenly realms.
>
> —EPHESIANS 6:11–12

This passage is also a reminder that God's children are not immune to spiritual attacks. If Satan can't take you out, he will try to wear you out. So you have to remain vigilant and make a conscious decision to partner with God to fight against even your own flesh nature, which is a weapon the enemy uses against you.

The decision to partner with God and submit to the

Holy Spirit is a daily decision we all have to make. John the Baptist said it best: "He [Jesus] must become greater; I must become less" (John 3:30).

CLOSING THE DOOR TO THE ENEMY

A life of obedience is the way to close the door to the enemy in our lives. The enemy tries to use our own sinful nature against us. But God has equipped us with everything we need to fight the good fight of faith against the attacks of the evil one. Jesus said, "Watch and pray so that you will not fall into temptation. The spirit is willing, but the flesh is weak" (Matt. 26:41). When you feel weak, cry out to your heavenly Father. He is here with you right now.

As we've seen from Scripture, God called each one of us to a particular purpose as we walk in a relationship with Him. Getting out of the cycle of the flesh and stepping into our purpose in Christ requires walking in surrender to God's will. This is what crucifying the flesh is all about. Paul says it this way in Galatians 5:24–25: "Those who belong to Christ Jesus have crucified the flesh with its passions and desires. Since we live by the Spirit, let us keep in step with the Spirit."

Historically, words such as *surrender* or *obedience* made my patients cringe—often because of misconceptions they held about God. Throughout the next few pages we will address the two most common misconceptions about God. Then we will talk about God's heart toward you.

MISCONCEPTION 1: THE DICTATOR

Many people shy away from letting God into their hearts because they see Him as a dictator. They believe that once they surrender their lives to Jesus, God will take away any freedom they may have, lock them into a box of rules, and throw away the keys. My friends, what you're thinking of is religion, not a relationship with God.

God is not a dictator. A dictator commands people to do things he's not willing to do himself. A dictator doesn't care about having a relationship with his followers. A dictator only cares about himself. Jesus is the one true God who came to earth willingly to die for His people so they may have eternal life with Him (John 3:16). In my search for truth as a Muslim, I looked up other religions. None of them offers what the gospel of Jesus Christ offers: *total freedom* from ever having to earn or achieve our way to anything.

Does this mean we can use our freedom to do whatever we want? No. Just like any good father, God knows what will hurt us and what will help us. But God is not going to expect us to get everything right as soon as we surrender our lives to Him. He knows we will struggle. In fact, He knew the exact struggles you would face after you gave your life to Him. Despite all that, God still says, "I choose you" (Eph. 1:4), "I am committed to you" (Phil. 1:6), "I am with you" (Matt. 28:20), and "I am for you" (Rom. 8:31).

MISCONCEPTION 2: THE HARSH JUDGE

Is God a judge? Absolutely. He is a righteous judge. By His standard of holiness we stood condemned. Yet, in Jesus, He showed us the extent of His love for us. In Jesus, God chose to pay the penalty of the judgment we deserved so that we can have a Father-child relationship with Him. So regardless of what your past looks like, regardless of the mistakes you've made, God is faithful to His Word. God promises that if we confess our sins to Him He will forgive us (1 John 1:9).

If you've read my books or heard me speak, you'll see that I use this verse often. This is because God's forgiveness is a hard concept to grasp, especially when we've been stuck on the hamster wheel of achievement for a long time. Our God is a forgiving Father. Forgiveness is a trait Jesus reflected so clearly on the cross. When we can't see past our brokenness, we keep ourselves from receiving the very healing God extends to us through a relationship with Him.

In the next chapter we'll look at the necessary steps to overcome being led by our own flesh. Until then, I invite you to hold on to this truth: God is the perfect Father. What He is extending to you is an invitation to let Him come into your life—every nook and crevice—and heal every part of you that has been wounded. God invites you to come to Him as you are, lay your defense mechanisms at the cross, and watch His miracle-working power breathe life into every part of you that you have given up on and transform it for His glory.

Questions for Reflection

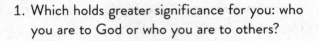

1. Which holds greater significance for you: who you are to God or who you are to others?

2. Do you care more about how God sees you or about how others see you?

3. Why do we struggle to prioritize God's perspective over people's opinions?

Chapter 10

YOUR BATTLE PLAN
AGAINST ENEMY 2

LAYING DOWN OUR defense mechanisms involves healing the hurt that's hidden behind those defense walls for so long. In this chapter we will go through the practical steps of laying down our defense mechanisms, uncovering our hurts, and receiving God's healing. We do this through what I call the forgiveness template.

Before we dive into the forgiveness template, let's look at the three types of forgiveness we need to extend. The first is *forgiving yourself* for your past mistakes. Listen: we've all messed up—some of us more than others. A lot of times we're willing to forgive other people, but we're not willing to forgive ourselves because we hold ourselves to a higher standard. Choosing not to forgive yourself opens the door to internal torment. I've held on to unforgiveness toward myself many times throughout my life, thinking it somehow held me accountable not to repeat the same mistake again. But in reality it just kept me stuck in a cycle of torment—the very cycle from which God was trying to set me free.

The Word of God says, "If the Son sets you free, you

will be free indeed" (John 8:36). Jesus extends this freedom to you. He died for your sins, past, present, and future. God is inviting you right now to experience the freedom He redeemed for you with His precious Son's blood. I pray you are willing to receive that freedom from your heavenly Father, who loves you, who forgives you, and whose mercies toward you are new every morning (Lam. 3:22–23).

The second type of forgiveness is *forgiving those who have hurt us*. This is one of the toughest ones to extend because sometimes the hurt runs deep. Oftentimes this hurt has been rooted in us from childhood, and we've covered it up with so many defense mechanisms we don't even know if we can reach down deep enough. Other times we don't want to uncover the hurt out of fear it will bring up emotions we have shut off.

Right now, ask the Lord to give you the grace you need to uncover the wound(s) in every nook and crevice of your soul, and allow His Holy Spirit to heal every wound that has been festering. I would never ask you to do something that 1) isn't biblical, and 2) I haven't done myself and seen work miracles in my own life.

My story of hurt may not be the same as yours, and I wish I could be sitting with you and listening to your story. But someone much better than I is with you right now. His name is the Holy Spirit, the Counselor, the Comforter, the best one to take you through the forgiveness process. It takes a lot of courage to step out and choose to forgive, but I promise you it's worth it!

The third type of unforgiveness is unpopular and rarely talked about in church. In fact, you may even shy away from admitting you have it because of the shame that's usually associated with it. I'm talking about *unforgiveness toward God.* In my years as a believer, I have found this to be the hardest one to admit because I felt as if I was accusing God of something and that admitting it would make Him mad at me. I'd like to share this story with you to help you better understand this concept.

ANGRY AT GOD

Through the years I've counseled many people who had experienced trauma in their lifetime. After a trauma it's typical to feel angry and confused at the injustice you experienced. At times I sensed that the person was holding a grudge against God. Whenever I'd ask, 99 percent of the time my patients would express feeling ashamed for holding such feelings. The problem, however, was that their shame kept them from releasing the anger they had— and as a result they remained tormented.

The situation usually went something like this: a patient would experience a traumatic event. The enemy, who is the author of confusion and the one behind chaos, would sweep in and whisper lies and doubt in the person's ear, similar to what he did to me (see my story in chapter 3). When demons have your attention, they whisper the same destructive lies over and over—anything that will make you doubt God's faithfulness and love for you, or anything that will attack your identity. So the best way to tackle the enemy's lies is by exposing them. To do it, I always go to the source of truth, the Holy Spirit.

"Don't you think God would be mad at me for telling Him I'm mad at Him?" a patient once asked me.

"He already knows you're mad at Him," I responded.

"And maybe He orchestrated for us to meet so you can finally bring it out in the open and process through your anger with Him."

"How do I do that?" she answered.

"Tell Him," I said.

"What?" she asked, shocked.

I'm going to tell you what I told her. God wants you to tell Him. The enemy wants nothing more than to keep you from the One who loves you most. First he whispers lies about Him; and then he convinces you to keep your anger in, knowing that as long as it's unresolved, you'll stay far from God so he (the devil) can keep tormenting you.

To resolve this issue, talk to God. If as you're reading this the Lord is reminding you about a grievance you're holding against Him, please talk to Him. Tell Him you're upset that He allowed XYZ to happen. Cry out to Him. Share your grief with Him. Whatever you do, don't stop talking to Him. The same way you'd want your child to talk with you to resolve an issue he has with you, talk to your Father and seek His face about the situation.

The reason it's so important you get with God to talk about grudges you may be holding against Him is that it's a chance to talk to the One who loves you most. It also short-circuits the enemy's plan to keep inserting lies and doubt about God because you're going straight to the source instead of replaying your experience over and over, trying to figure it out on your own. Holding it all in gives the enemy ample opportunity to add his own two cents about the situation.

ANSWER HIS CALL

As you're reading this, if you feel God nudge your heart to process through unforgiveness you hold toward Him, please answer His call. He is extending His hand to you, to heal you. You don't have to say an elaborate prayer. All you need to do is speak from your heart the way Jesus once cried out to the Father in desperation: "My God, my God, why have You forsaken me?"

Does this mean God will give you the answer you want? No. But the fact remains that He made you. He loves you. He knows how to talk to you and give you the peace you're seeking.

Again, does this mean God will give you the answer you want? No. But remember: *He made you, He loves you, and He knows how to talk to you and give you the peace you're seeking.*

We're about to go over the forgiveness template where you will get a chance to process through your own hurts with God—whether they are resentments you hold against yourself, against others, or against God. The goal of this process is to get them out so you can experience the healing that only comes from God.

Before we start the forgiveness process, I want to give you a visual of how unforgiveness usually takes place so that in the future you'll be able to discern unprocessed hurt and process through it before it goes any further.

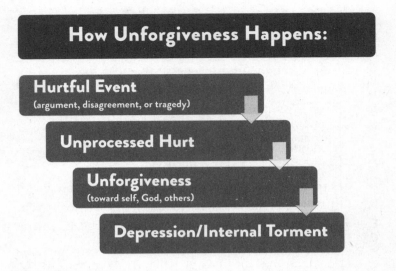

Usually by the time someone comes in to see me for counseling, they've been living in step 4 of this diagram—sometimes for decades. I'm not saying that every hurtful event leads to depression and anxiety, but I've seen how unprocessed hurt does. Before we know it, we are carrying unforgiveness. God didn't make our hearts to bear the weight of unforgiveness. Unforgiveness is heavy, and it drains the life out of us. Think of someone in your life who keeps records of what this or that person did to hurt them. There's no way that person is joyful. They are likely tormented with depression.

I have worked with patients who've tried all types of medication to resolve their depression and anxiety, only to conclude that it was a direct result of unresolved hurt they needed to process. So I walked my patients through the act of surrendering their pain to the One who can heal them—God.

I know the words *surrender* and *forgiveness* can be

dreaded words, especially in the Christian community, believe it or not. And I truly believe those words are dreaded because they've been misused by people in the church community. So many patients have told me they were made to forgive a perpetrator without processing the hurt they endured by that perpetrator. This further victimized my patients. Condemning someone into forgiving somebody else, or trying to guilt-trip them into forgiveness, will drive that person into further depression and further away from God.

What produces true healing is walking someone through *how to forgive* properly. It means showing someone that God does not condone abuse. God does not condone sin. God does not turn His face away from violence and pretend it didn't happen. That is not the God we serve!

Does this mean God condones unforgiveness? No. He wants us to live a life marked by forgiveness. He also knows He is the only One able to heal our hurts. That's why He invites us to come to Him (Matt. 11:28–30). You see, Jesus is acquainted with every type of pain we could ever imagine because He felt it. Hebrews 4:14–16 says,

> Therefore, since we have a great high priest who has ascended into heaven, Jesus the Son of God, let us hold firmly to the faith we profess. For we do not have a high priest who is unable to empathize with our weaknesses, but we have one who has been tempted in every way, just as we are—yet he did not sin. Let us then approach God's throne of grace with confidence, so that we may receive mercy and find grace to help us in our time of need.

Jesus knows every painful event you have gone through. He wants you to bring it to Him and trust that He can heal you.

Patients often prefer counselors who have gone through something similar to what they went through. This is because we all want to feel heard and understood, and we believe that a person who has gone through something similar to what we experienced is more likely to understand us and empathize with us. That person is more likely to provide us with the encouragement we need at the time we need it. That person will also be acquainted with our pain and know the path to get us out of it, because they've walked it themselves.

Jesus, our Wonderful Counselor (Isa. 9:6), experienced every possible pain you can imagine. Jesus was betrayed by one of His close friends, and that betrayal led ultimately to His sentencing and death. Are you dealing with the pain of betrayal? Perhaps you shared something close and personal with a friend or family member, and they betrayed your trust by spreading rumors about you. Or maybe you trusted a business partner, just to find out they went behind your back and betrayed you. Rest assured, Jesus knows the pain of betrayal.

He knows how it feels to be abandoned. He spent years with His disciples; yet when He was arrested, they all went their separate ways, and one of His closest friends denied even knowing Him.

Right now, if you're dealing with the pain of someone you love not being there for you physically and/or emotionally, Jesus knows your pain. His own family thought He was crazy and tried to get Him arrested (Mark 3:21). It's one thing for an acquaintance not to believe in us, but when a close friend or family member doesn't, the hurt goes deep. Jesus is acquainted with that hurt.

Jesus was familiar with the pain of rejection. Throughout His ministry, religious leaders accused Him of casting out demons by the power of the devil (Matt. 12:22–32; Luke 11:14–23). And when their accusations didn't lead anywhere, they rejected Him as the Messiah and yelled out, "Crucify him!" (Luke 23:21).

Jesus knew the pain of being mocked (Mark 14:65). As He was beaten, the soldiers spit in His face and made fun of Him. Jesus was also well acquainted with abuse. He was beaten repeatedly (Matt. 26:67). The Bible says that the soldiers plucked out pieces of His beard while making fun of Him and put a crown of thorns on His head. Yet when they crucified Him, Jesus said, "Father, forgive them, for they do not know what they are doing" (Luke 23:34). Was Jesus excusing His perpetrators' behavior? No. Jesus was reflecting the heart of God, forgiving.

FORGIVENESS DOES NOT REQUIRE RECONCILIATION

Before we proceed, let me make something clear. Forgiving someone and choosing to reconcile with them are two totally separate issues. When Jesus died on the cross for us, God extended forgiveness toward us. But we were not reconciled to God until we turned away from our sin, turned to God, repented of our sins, and received Jesus as our Lord and Savior.

The same principle applies to people. Just because you forgive someone for what they have done does not mean you need to reconcile and condone further abuse from the person. Forgiveness says, "I choose to forgive you for what you did." Reconciliation may only happen when the person has displayed repentance for their actions through changed behavior over a period of time.

As I said before, attempting to forgive someone without processing through the hurt they caused us leads to a superficial type of forgiveness, which is no forgiveness at all. It is *only* when we process through the hurt and are honest with God about the pain the offender caused that we're able to move forward in forgiveness.

When I teach on forgiveness, I bring two shredders and a set of flashcards with me. I set up shredders on each side of the church altar and have flashcards placed on every seat in the congregation. I conclude my message of forgiveness with a response time song. This allows people time to talk with God about their hurts, write down their grievances, forgive, and finally shred the piece of paper. This signifies that they have chosen to forgive their hurts and move forward.

Although I am not with you in person as you step into the forgiveness process, please know that I have prayed the following prayer over you:

> *Faithful Father, I pray that my brother or sister in Christ will feel Your tangible presence around them. I pray that Your presence will shield their minds from any doubt that may come their way. I pray that Your love will encompass them, that they'll feel comfortable opening up their hearts to You and pouring out their hurts to You, knowing You care about every detail of their lives. I pray that You will*

show up mightily in their lives. I pray they'll see You as their defender and strong tower. Lord, I pray they will feel Your grace through each and every step. I pray they will come out of this process healed and confident that You who began a good work in them will bring it to completion. I pray that You will order their steps according to Your will. Thank You, Father, that You hear our prayers. In Jesus' name, amen.

THE FORGIVENESS TEMPLATE (SAMPLE):

1. Whenever I go through the forgiveness template in my life, I imagine myself in a courtroom. I imagine God, who is also my Father, as the judge. This gives me peace that He is for me. I imagine my offender on the other side as the defendant and myself as the prosecutor. Then I plead my case to my Father using the next steps.

2. Identify and write down the offender's name and tell God what the person did to you. For example: "Father, Mary betrayed my trust when she shared things that I told her in confidence. I'm so mad at her. Father, I don't think I could ever be friends with her again!"

3. Do not make excuses for the person. Talk to God honestly. Let all your emotions out and allow room for God to respond to you.

4. Tell God, "I choose to forgive Mary for (the offense)."

THE FORGIVENESS TEMPLATE:

1. Approach God confidently, knowing He cares for you.

2. Identify and write down the offender's name and tell God what the person did to you. (Refer to the above template for an example.)

3. Do not make excuses for the person. Talk to God honestly. Let all your emotions out and allow room for God to respond to you.

4. Tell God, "I choose to forgive [name] for [the offense]."

Please use this template until you memorize the steps of forgiveness. The reality is, offenses will come because we live in a sinful world; but when we make a commitment to live a life marked by forgiveness, the enemy won't be able to get a foothold in our lives, no matter how much he tries. At that point we would be living out James 4:7, which says, "Submit yourselves, then, to God. Resist the devil, and he will flee from you."

QUESTIONS FOR REFLECTION

One of the most difficult steps I've come across with patients is helping them identify their own emotions. About 70 percent of the time we circle around "mad" and "numb." The former is a *fight response* that gives us the illusion of control, whereas the latter is a *flight response* that seeks to deny the reality of the hurt. Until something triggers it, that is! Since I'm not with you in person, I've listed twenty of the most common emotions that result from unprocessed hurt. It is so important that you identify which emotion(s) the hurt caused so you're able to let go of them when you forgive the person.

Emotions that stem from unprocessed hurt:

anxious, out of control, betrayed, rejected, unsafe, violated, alone, confused, stranded, sad, helpless, guilty, ashamed, condemned, inferior, unwanted, jealous, cheated, scared, incompetent

Name	Offense	How you felt as a result of the offense
Example: Mary Smith	*She gossiped and spread lies about me to my friends.*	**I felt** *betrayed*
		I felt
		I felt
		I felt
		I felt
		I felt

In what ways have you experienced the Holy Spirit during this process?

PART III
ENEMY 3— THE WORLD

Chapter 11

PUTTING FAITH IN PEOPLE RATHER THAN GOD

I F SATAN CAN'T convince you to put your faith in him or in yourself, he will convince you to put your faith in others. This leads us to enemy 3—the world. In this section we will focus on how placing our faith in people rather than God can lead us down a path of destruction. The Bible is filled with passages that advise against putting our faith in people, along with the consequences of doing so. Here are a few examples:

> Don't put your confidence in powerful people; there is no help for you there. When they breathe their last, they return to the earth, and all their plans die with them. But joyful are those who have the God of Israel as their helper, whose hope is in the LORD their God.
>
> —PSALM 146:3–5, NLT

> It is better to take refuge in the LORD than to trust in humans.
>
> —PSALM 118:8

God wants our faith to be grounded in Him alone. Anytime our faith is divided between God and man, we enter troubled waters. Before we jump into how putting our faith in people can affect our lives negatively, let's take a look at how it affected Solomon's. Using Scripture, we will examine King Solomon's life and see exactly how the man once known as the wisest to ever live became entrapped in the destructive cycle of the world.

Of course, this didn't happen overnight. In the beginning of his reign Solomon was fully surrendered to God. In fact, during his first year as king, Solomon had a dream in which God said, "Ask for whatever you want me to give you" (1 Kings 3:5). Solomon replied, "So give your servant a discerning heart to govern your people and to distinguish between right and wrong" (1 Kings 3:9). In other words, Solomon asked God for wisdom so he could lead the people well. Throughout the next few pages we're going to dive into the subtle cycle that changed Solomon from a wise and God-fearing king into a cynical, miserable, and idolatrous monarch who is unrecognizable from his former self.

STEP 1: DECEPTION

Throughout the years of his reign Solomon turned away from his *full* commitment to God and compromised his values to please others. We often fall into deception when we believe we can please God and man at the same time, or when we try to keep one foot in the world and one foot with God, while walking the straight and narrow path. That's impossible. The world sways you one way while God says, "Follow Me," in another direction. That's why a decision must be made in your life: to follow man's way or Jesus' way.

Long before Solomon, God set the standard by saying, "You shall have no other gods before me" (Exod. 20:3). This is because you and I were created to worship God. When we choose not to be fully devoted to God, our interests become divided. Soon after that, instead of looking up to the One who made us, we start looking around for answers.

Solomon fell into the deception that he could secure life's satisfaction from what was directly in front of him. First Kings 11:1–10 says,

> King Solomon, however, loved many foreign women besides Pharaoh's daughter—Moabites, Ammonites, Edomites, Sidonians and Hittites. They were from nations about which the LORD had told the Israelites, "You must not intermarry with them, because they will surely turn your hearts after their gods." Nevertheless, Solomon held fast to them in love. He had seven hundred wives of royal birth and three hundred concubines, and his wives led him astray. As Solomon grew old, his wives turned his heart after other gods, and his heart was not fully devoted to the LORD his God, as the heart of David his father had been. He followed Ashtoreth the goddess of the Sidonians, and Molek the detestable god of the Ammonites. So Solomon did evil in the eyes of the LORD; he did not follow the LORD completely, as David his father had done. On a hill east of Jerusalem, Solomon built a high place for

Chemosh the detestable god of Moab, and for Molek the detestable god of the Ammonites. He did the same for all his foreign wives, who burned incense and offered sacrifices to their gods. The LORD became angry with Solomon because his heart had turned away from the LORD, the God of Israel, who had appeared to him twice. Although he had forbidden Solomon to follow other gods, Solomon did not keep the LORD's command.

The previous passage marks Solomon's entrance into step 1—the deceptive cycle of the world. From what we see in this passage, Solomon's desire to please his wives outgrew his desire to please God. The Bible never says that Solomon was not devoted to God. It says that he was not devoted to God *fully*. So you see where the deception is. The world wants to deceive us into believing we can have one foot in God's kingdom and one foot in the world. But before we know it our interests are divided. Our values are compromised. And we begin to serve creation rather than the Creator.

STEP 2: DISAPPOINTMENTS

Solomon had everything from a worldly standpoint, only to reach the latter years of his life and say, "I have seen all the things that are done under the sun; all of them are meaningless, a chasing after the wind" (Eccles. 1:14).

Solomon's disappointments are clearly laid out in Ecclesiastes 2:3–11:

I tried cheering myself with wine, and embracing folly—my mind still guiding me with wisdom.

I wanted to see what was good for people to do under heaven during the few days of their lives. I undertook great projects: I built houses for myself and planted vineyards. I made gardens and parks and planted all kinds of fruit trees in them. I made reservoirs to water groves of flourishing trees. I bought male and female slaves and had other slaves who were born in my house. I also owned more herds and flocks than anyone in Jerusalem before me. I amassed silver and gold for myself, and the treasure of kings and provinces. I acquired male and female singers, and a harem as well—the delights of a man's heart. I became greater by far than anyone in Jerusalem before me. In all this my wisdom stayed with me. I denied myself nothing my eyes desired; I refused my heart no pleasure. My heart took delight in all my labor, and this was the reward for all my toil. Yet when I surveyed all that my hands had done and what I had toiled to achieve, everything was meaningless, a chasing after the wind; nothing was gained under the sun.

Here Solomon is presenting to us the rulebook of what *not* to do. He is saying, "Look, I have done everything I thought would bring me happiness. I ventured off and tried everything the world has to offer, just to find it meaningless."

STEP 3: DEPRESSION

Had Solomon walked into a therapist's office today and verbalized the despair he expresses throughout Ecclesiastes,

I can assure you he would have been diagnosed with clinical depression.

Let's take a closer look at the diagnosis of major depressive disorder and examine how King Solomon would have fit the profile for it today. According to the National Institute of Mental Health, major depressive disorder, also known as MDD, is one of the most common clinical diagnoses in the field of mental health, affecting an estimated 21 million adults in the United States each year.[1] Per the *Diagnostic and Statistical Manual* (DSM-5), this type of clinical depression is indicated when someone has experienced five or more symptoms during the same two-week period. Let's go over each symptom and compare it to the biblical accounts of Solomon's statements in Ecclesiastes.

1. The first symptom of clinical depression is showing a *depressed mood* most of the day, nearly every day. Ecclesiastes 2:17–18 records Solomon expressing grief and disappointment with life. He said, "So I hated life, because the work that is done under the sun was grievous to me. All of it is meaningless, a chasing after the wind. I hated all the things I had toiled for under the sun, because I must leave them to the one who comes after me."

2. The second symptom is a *markedly diminished interest or pleasure in activities*. In his later years Solomon referred to his life as *meaningless* and the achievements he normally would have taken pleasure in as *meaningless*. Ecclesiastes 2:11 says, "Yet when I surveyed all that my hands had done and what I had toiled to achieve, everything was meaningless, a chasing after the wind; nothing was gained under the sun." A few verses later, he said, "So I hated life, because the work that is done under the sun

was grievous to me. All of it is meaningless, a chasing after the wind" (v. 17).

3. Another well-known symptom of clinical depression is *fatigue or loss of energy* over a period of weeks. Solomon said, "...I have poured my effort and skill under the sun. This too is meaningless. So my heart began to despair over all my toilsome labor under the sun" (Eccles. 2:19–20).

4. You don't have to look far into Ecclesiastes to spot Solomon's *feelings of worthlessness,* marking another symptom of clinical depression. In Ecclesiastes 1:2 he said, "'Meaningless! Meaningless!' says the Teacher. 'Utterly meaningless! Everything is meaningless.'" A few verses later he said, "No one remembers the former generations, and even those yet to come will not be remembered by those who follow them" (v. 11). Then, in Ecclesiastes 7:15, he continued, "In this meaningless life of mine I have seen both of these: the righteous perishing in their righteousness, and the wicked living long in their wickedness."

5. Last, it's clear from Solomon's thought process that he had been having *recurrent thoughts of death* as he surveyed his life and works. In Ecclesiastes 2:18 he said, "I hated all the things I had toiled for under the sun, because I must leave them to the one who comes after me." In Ecclesiastes 3:19–20 he continued, "Surely the fate of human beings is like that of the animals; the same fate awaits them both: As one dies, so dies the other. All have the same breath; humans have no advantage over animals. Everything is meaningless. All go to the same place; all come from dust, and to dust all return." Toward the end of Ecclesiastes he said, "For the living know that they will die, but the dead know nothing; they have no further reward, and even their name is forgotten" (Eccles. 9:5).

You may read this and be tempted to think, "Well, I'm nothing like Solomon. It's not like I'm building statues anywhere or worshipping other gods." In reality, as we will see throughout the following chapters, it doesn't take building a statue to not be fully committed to God. What usually sways us from being fully devoted to God are small missteps here and there.

Solomon's life is a fitting example of how one decision after another outside of God's will can lead us to a state of despair—the state where we feel as if nothing and no one can console us. The state where we've looked everywhere for a solution, and all our efforts are futile: "chasing after the wind," as Solomon put it. The world is full of false promises that aim to get us to fall into its destructive cycle. To recap, the cycle is:

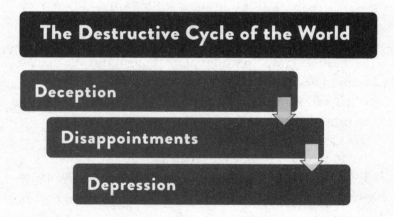

The Destructive Cycle of the World

Deception

Disappointments

Depression

In the next chapter we're going to look at a few different cases in which people, like Solomon, fell into the destructive cycle of the world, resulting in depression-related symptoms.

QUESTIONS FOR REFLECTION

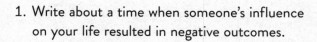

1. Write about a time when someone's influence on your life resulted in negative outcomes.

2. Looking back, what were some red flags in your friendship/relationship with that person?

Chapter 12

THE REALM OF
THE WORLD

FOR OUR DIVE into depression-related symptoms, I'd like to use real examples from people's lives. My hope is that one will resonate with you and show you how easy it is to fall into this trap. I hope this will not only encourage you to remain vigilant and guard your heart but also show you the hope that is available in case you are entrapped in this cycle.

CASE 1: THE HERO COMPLEX

Stephen was a thirty-five-year-old male who presented to therapy with symptoms of depression. Well-established in his career, he said he had just gotten out of a relationship where he felt taken advantage of financially by his ex-girlfriend. When asked what brought him to therapy, he replied, "For as long as I can remember, I keep falling for women who just mooch from me. I get tired of it. I start to resent them. I shut down, end the relationship, and end up forking over the bill to move them out. I'm tired of this!" Stephen came to therapy at the advice of his parents.

As we dug into his childhood, Stephen said his parents divorced when he was about twelve, and his mother, whom he lived with, remarried. He said she and his stepdad started a new family, and he felt left out most of the time. He mentioned that he and his mother had grown close between the divorce and her remarrying to the point where he became her confidant. He said he liked that role because it made him feel special and dependable.

When he entered adulthood, he continued to play the same role in his relationships. Although being needed gave him the sense of security he wanted in the relationship, after a while he grew resentful because he gave without getting anything in return from his girlfriends. This resulted in disappointment and depression.

Through therapy Stephen discovered his pattern was born out of his attempts to avoid the pain of rejection. He learned he had been trying to re-create the close relationship he once had with his mom in his current relationships. He also learned he should not have been placed in the position of a confidant as a child. Throughout the steps I will go over with you, Stephen was able to stop the destructive cycle, stand on the assurance of God's love for him, and learn how to develop a healthy relationship with a significant other.

CASE 2: DEPENDENT PERSONALITY DISORDER

Mia came in with symptoms that indicated she had dependent personality disorder. This disorder is very hard to treat because it requires significant change in the patient's personality makeup, including her thought process that resulted in her current lifestyle behaviors. This is why personality disorders often carry a stigma of being hard to treat.

As I worked with Mia, it became clear that her dependent traits—though fitting the criteria for a dependent personality disorder—were merely patterns she learned to use from an incredibly young age. Mia was a very bright woman in her late twenties. Her father had passed away at an early age, and ever since then she and her mom had leaned on each other for support.

Through the years Mia met someone, they began dating, and eventually they married. Mia and her husband argued a lot the first few years of their marriage, which is typical as a married couple learns to adjust to their new life. As their arguments worsened through the years, however, Mia's husband threatened to separate. This led Mia to come in for therapy.

When asked about the issues surrounding her marriage, Mia mentioned that her husband and her mom didn't get along. Mia said, "My husband is jealous of my relationship with Mom." The more I worked with Mia, the more evident it became that her attachment with her mother was unhealthy. Mia sought her mom's input prior to making most of her decisions. In some instances it would have been more appropriate for Mia to call her husband and talk to him about a decision; instead she called her mom, which created further friction in her marriage.

Throughout our work together, Mia was able to see that her relationship with her mom had reached the point of codependency, a level that would not even have been appropriate in her relationship with her husband. Mia understood that the only person we are supposed to be codependent on is God and that God's order for relationships is for the spouse to take the second place, and then children, and so on. As I worked with Mia on the steps I will go over with you later in this book, she was able to reclaim her identity in Christ and reprioritize her relationships in a way that allowed her and her husband to grow together in unity and her and her mom to have a healthy relationship.

CASE 3: PEOPLE PLEASER

Simon grew up in a tight-knit family. They always placed one another first and often preached "blood is thicker than water," as Simon said. During his teenage years Simon worked in the family business and was happy doing so. In his early twenties he felt a call from God to switch careers. His family became furious. Soon after, Simon was faced with the decision either to move forward with what he believed God wanted him to do and face his dad's wrath, as he referred to it, or continue to walk in his family's plans for his life. This included his taking over the family business one day. Over the next few years he kept working in the family business to please his father and not "ruffle any feathers," as he said. Eventually Simon began to feel dissatisfied with his life. He no longer enjoyed the work he was doing. He felt hopeless and helpless, all of which are symptoms of major depressive disorder, by the way.

Simon's depression stemmed from not walking in the plans and purposes his heavenly Father had laid out for him. In therapy I worked with him on strengthening his relationship with God—a crucial step we will cover later in the book. As he grew closer to God, he felt more confident in the direction toward which God was calling him. He understood the true meaning of Psalm 37:4: "Take delight in the LORD, and he will give you the desires of your heart."

This speaks to the fact that God places His desires for our lives within us, and we are to live out His desires. Simon was able to assert himself with the family members who objected to his leaving the family business. His faith grew as he watched God provide for him in many ways. Simon regained his sense of joy and clung to his faith in the Lord.

CASE 4: FLATTERER

Patricia was the number one salesperson in her company and proud of maintaining that record for four years in a row. During our first therapy session she complimented almost every piece in my office. This included the therapeutic techniques listed in my profile and the school I attended, among other things. When she walked out of the office, she was charming and overly complimentary to our staff. I could see she was very likable. The question was, How could such a likable, charming person be so depressed?

You see, from an early age Patricia learned, "If I can get this person to like me, then I'll be safe." She continued in this pattern throughout her life. It was even positively reinforced in her career as she received awards and recognition for being the top salesperson. Flattery, however, didn't fix the yearning she had deep down for a sense of safety. She felt enslaved to a pattern and didn't know how to get out of it.

I worked with Patricia on understanding who she was in Christ and making that the foundation of her identity and security. It took a little while for this to work in her life because she had been living in the other cycle for years. But, as Hebrews 4:12 says, "For the word of God is alive and active. Sharper than any double-edged sword, it penetrates even to dividing soul and spirit, joints and marrow; it judges the thoughts and attitudes of the heart." By spending time with God, Patricia found that His Word penetrated through the lies and fears with which she had been living. Using the concepts we will cover in chapter 15, she gained assurance of who she is in Christ and reflected that identity in her lifestyle.

CASE 5: THE WRONG FOUNDATION

A patient came in for therapy after the loss of her mom. Throughout her grief treatment my patient described herself with words such as *shattered* and sentences like "I feel as if I don't know who I am or what my purpose is in life." The longer I worked with her, the clearer it became that she had built her life upon the wrong foundation— her mother.

Moving forward after losing someone you love is hard enough. But when your sense of self has hinged on the person you lost it makes your grief even worse. Healing from this grief requires major identity renovation. It's like going into a house that was built on a broken foundation, uprooting the house, setting it on the right foundation, and then fixing all the internal damage caused by the house being set on the wrong foundation.

In this case, the house was my patient's sense of self. The broken foundation was her mom. Helping my patient rebuild her identity required her to follow the process we will go over at the end of this book.

As we've discovered through this chapter, temptation to put our faith in people is everywhere, and falling into this temptation carries with it mental and spiritual consequences. Proverbs 4:23 says, "Above all else, guard your heart, for everything you do flows from it." The steps we will go through in chapter 15 will help you do just that.

QUESTIONS FOR REFLECTION

1. Which of the stories in this chapter resonated with you?

2. Why?

Chapter 13

DESTRUCTIVE PATTERNS OF BEHAVIOR

WHEN WE AREN'T fully committed to God, we engage in patterns of behavior to maintain our relationships with the objects of our faith—in this case, people. These patterns of behavior may give us a false sense of security in the short term. In reality, they just keep us trapped in the very cycle from which Jesus came to set us free. Let's look at them now.

People-pleasing: a form of self-betrayal where we aim to please someone at our own expense.

On the surface, this behavior may mask itself as a selfless, "Christian" act. But people-pleasing is rooted in a sense of identity that isn't secure in God's love. So we aim to gain this security by earning acceptance from others. People-pleasing can include turning your back on your own values to say yes to the person you're trying to please. Whenever I've treated people who struggle with people-pleasing, instead of telling them to stop doing it, I tried to figure out why they were doing it. Nine times out of ten we take this approach because we are insecure in God's love for us. We're trying to please others either to get them to like us or to prevent them from disliking us because it gives us a false sense of security. This behavior typically starts at an early age when the people we are trying to please are our source of security.

One of my patients grew up with a parent who struggled with alcohol. When the parent was intoxicated, my patient knew she had to agree with the parent and walk on eggshells around them to avoid confrontation. At the time, disagreeing with the parent—who was her only source of security—would have threatened her safety. If your childhood experience was like this one, I am so sorry.

I've also come across many patients who had to mediate between their divorced parents because the parents refused to get along. The child was stuck between pleasing Mom and pleasing Dad. They were so used to this pattern that they carried it over into adulthood; they even viewed their relationship with God this way. This put them on the striving bandwagon. God wants us to be set free from this pattern. He wants us to be concerned only about pleasing Him, and we do this by remaining in Him (John 15).

I'm not saying to remain in Christ because it sounds hyper-spiritual. I'm telling you this out of experience, both personally and professionally. Whenever I don't fill myself with God's truth about who I am, I start to feel burned out, and it shows in both my thought life and my actions.

Here's an analogy to explain this process. Think of yourself as a plant. God is the water. The world is the sun. Spending time with God is like watering the plant. God gave you the sun (people in your life). If you subject the plant to the sun without water, it may survive for a little while, but after a couple of days it's going to get burned. That's what happens to you and me when we don't spend time with God. Our spirits are not made to thrive without

God. We may try, and it may last a little while. But deep down we will always feel like something is missing until we turn back to the One who loves us beyond measure—our heavenly Father.

On the other hand, if you keep a plant away from the sun yet give it water, it will do well, but not as well as it would have had it been in the sun. This is why having people to do life with is beneficial to our walk with Christ. People aren't God, but God can certainly use people as His hands and feet to help us accomplish His will in our lives.

If you struggle with people-pleasing, the following steps are intended to help you overcome this destructive pattern of behavior.

1. Spend time with God and allow Him to fill you with truths about who you are in Him. Let God dictate your identity, not the world or other people. At times you may say no to someone who does not like boundaries, and that person may retaliate. That does not mean you should see yourself in a negative light because of that one person or group of people who didn't respect you anyway.

2. Resist the temptation to say yes to a commitment right away. This was one of the hardest things for me to learn because I like to give definitive answers, and I like to get closure for things. So I felt that not saying yes or no right away left something hanging over my head until I made a decision. Or it made me feel indecisive at the moment and look bad to the person who was asking me for a favor. Resisting the temptation to answer right away gives us the chance to check in with ourselves to see if this is something we want to do. This will also keep us from saying yes to something, regretting it, then not showing up and feeling guilty for not showing up. Now we're beating ourselves up because we just backed out of a commitment.

So the next time someone asks you to help out with something or asks you to commit to an event, try saying, "Thank you for thinking of me. Let me think about it, and I'll let you know by (tomorrow, next week, next month)." If you decide not to accept the offer, say something like, "Thanks again for thinking of me, but I'm not going to do XYZ this time."

3. Get in the habit of asking God, "Father, is this opportunity from You?" Again, I'm not trying to sound hyper-spiritual here. But so many opportunities will come your way in life that seem good when actually they create a distraction from where God wants you to be. At the end of the day, we are here for God's plans and purposes, to do His will, as it says in Ephesians 2:10. So our time here is for God to direct, not for people to direct. That's why you want to get in the habit of asking God, "Is this opportunity from You?" This habit will help you if you're around people who guilt you into doing things that seem spiritual yet drain the life out of you.

This is especially true if you feel burned out from doing ministry work but feel guilty saying no. If this describes a situation you're in, remember your ministry is never supposed to supersede the ministry that's before your eyes—that is, your spouse and children. They are your primary ministry. If you find yourself burned out, please go to your heavenly Father and ask Him, "Is this from You?" Jesus is the Prince of Peace (Isa. 9:6). That means if the decision is from God, He will give you peace about it. If it isn't, you will not feel at rest.

Compromise: being swayed from the truth due to

lacking proper discernment where people are concerned. Compromise stems from a lack of proper reverence for God and His Word. If we don't spend enough time with God and anchor ourselves in His Word, we will be easily led astray.

A couple of months ago my son and I were swimming in a lazy river. After we went around and around, we reached a point where we both wanted to get out. I told my son to hold on to me because the current was too strong for him to try to get out on his own. Other parents were giving the same instruction to their children. If their children didn't listen, the current swept them in the opposite direction. Then they had to keep going until they reached the next exit point.

The same concept applies to our relationship with God. Our Father knows the current of the world is too strong for us to overcome in our own strength. That's why the Bible puts great emphasis on keeping our eyes on Jesus, the author and finisher of our faith (Heb. 12:2, NKJV).

The world is filled with distractions that give us false promises and aim to sway us away from our walk with God. This is why we must remain in constant communication with our Father through the Holy Spirit. God's Word promises that if we need wisdom about something we must ask Him and He will give it to us freely without rebuke (Jas. 1:5). So if you're unsure about something, ask God.

As we walk closely with our Father, keeping our eyes on Him, He will order our steps according to His plans and purposes for our lives. It's a step-by-step process. God is not going to give us the whole plan because the goal is a relationship with Him marked by daily conversations.

It's clear from the biblical accounts of Solomon's life that he had lost sight of how important it is to consult with God on every matter, whether small or large. When we loosen our commitment to God, we act on our own limited understanding rather than wisdom from above.

The following is an exercise to help you discern your possible risk of falling into the trap of compromise. You must decide: Are you in Christ, or are you in the world? You can't be in both.

Take inventory of your social circle. The closer someone is to you, the more influence they likely have over your decisions (repeat for every person in your social circle).

- Name

- Are they drawing you closer to Jesus?

On our own, you and I are not strong enough to fight against the current of the culture that aims to get the gospel of Jesus to fit its own agenda. But in Christ we can live out 1 John 4:4: "You, dear children, are from God and have overcome them, because the one who is in you is greater than the one who is in the world."

As we walk with Christ, God will equip us to discern His will and enable us to stand firm in the face of cultural shifts. We know that culture is ever changing, but God's Word never changes. In Jesus we can keep journeying through this life, knowing the hope that awaits us in eternity with our Father. We know nothing in this world can satisfy us the way Jesus does. God created us with a yearning that only He can satisfy. We can go around and around looking for what might satisfy us only to conclude that nothing can come close to the presence of God and the joy that comes from His presence (Ps. 16:11).

Flattery: unlike blessing someone with compliments, flattery is rooted in selfish ambition.

When you flatter someone, you do it with the goal of getting someone to look favorably on you. Flattery is a form of emotional manipulation. It preys on people's need for acceptance. When it comes to flattery, you want to watch for it in the following two ways: being the victim of flattery and playing the role of the flatterer.

Make sure you don't fall prey to someone's flattery; you can do this by rooting your identity in Christ. When you know who you are in Christ, you will discern when someone's compliments are attached to selfish motives. God will give you the discernment you need for that moment. This is especially something to watch for if your love language[1] is words of affirmation. My primary love language certainly is, and I've learned to pray for discernment when someone gives me a series of compliments to make sure the person is not just trying to get me to like them.

The Bible says, "Do nothing out of selfish ambition or vain conceit. Rather, in humility value others above yourselves, not looking to your own interests but each of you to the interests of the others" (Phil. 2:3–4). This includes flattering people to gain something from them. Flattering people is a behavior learned at an early age. If you struggle with this, just know that reversing this habit will take some work on your part. Often we get into this habit to try to meet our need for security. As children of God, our security lies in our heavenly Father's ability to provide for us. God knows exactly what we need, and as we walk with Him, we develop trust that He will meet our needs accordingly.

Flattery is not loving to our neighbors or to our brothers and sisters in Christ. God wants our love for one another to be genuine. He wants us to reflect the love He showed us unto others, that they may come to know Him someday. Jesus said, "A new command I give you: Love one another. As I have loved you, so you must love one another" (John 13:34). This love can only be reflected when we have formed a healthy attachment with God, one in which our sense of security rests on His unshakable character.

God put us here on earth as ambassadors for Him (2 Cor. 5:20), meaning we are here to reflect Him to a world that doesn't know Him. As ambassadors for Christ, we are to love our brothers and sisters and strangers as He loves us. Once we rest secure in Him and know He meets our needs, as He says He does in Philippians 4:19, we will no longer have to flatter others for our own selfish gain.

If flattery is something you struggle with, it's not by accident you're reading this. God wants to set you free from flattery. So I encourage you, friend, to repent of it. Repentance means to turn your back on something—in this case, flattery—and to turn toward Jesus. Following are the steps to renouncing flattery from your life:

1. Confess it to God by saying something such as, "Faithful Father, I confess I've used flattery many times to get my way. I confess that this is sinful and I do it out of my own selfish ambition. I renounce using flattery to gain my own interests, whether it is at the expense of others or not. You are the God of truth, and You desire truth. Help me to worship You in spirit and in truth, to live a life that is pleasing to You. Thank You for Your grace and mercy that cover me. Most of all, thank You for Your forgiveness that is in Jesus Christ. Amen."

2. Ask God to remind you of who you are in Him and enable you to love people the way He loves them.

3. Thank God for forgiving you and resist the enemy when he tempts you to flatter others. The Bible says, "Submit yourselves, then, to God. Resist the devil, and he will flee from you" (Jas. 4:7).

At the root of each one of the above-mentioned patterns of behavior is our attempt to place a person in a role that only God should have in our lives. If you feel that you've drifted from allowing God to be God in your life, I encourage you to recommit to seeking Him and trusting Him for your needs. God is the best Father you could ever imagine. Regardless of how great a father you've had or how terrible or absent your dad may have been, God is the *only* Father who can satisfy your heart's yearning. He created you for a relationship with Him. It is only through a healthy relationship with your heavenly Father that you will no longer feel that something is missing in your life. And you will know He is the One you've been yearning for your whole life.

QUESTIONS FOR REFLECTION

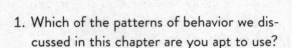

1. Which of the patterns of behavior we discussed in this chapter are you apt to use?

2. Choose two behavioral patterns from the ones we discussed: people-pleasing, compromise, flattery. In your notebook write about a recent instance when you used each one.

First Instance:

- Thinking back, why do you believe you used this pattern of behavior?

- What would've been a healthy long-term way to address and resolve the problem?

Second Instance:

- Thinking back, why do you believe you used this pattern of behavior?

- What would've been a healthy long-term way to address and resolve the problem?

Chapter 14

VICTORY OVER
EXTERNAL INFLUENCE

THROUGHOUT THE OLD Testament we read one story after another of God pursuing mankind, rescuing people, and teaching them to do right, just for them to turn right around and fall into the same trap of allowing the culture they lived in to seep into their hearts, leading them astray. Every now and then a person would remain faithful regardless of the cultural current he faced.

PATTERNS TELL A STORY

When it comes to studying human behavior, a big factor I look for is patterns. People's patterns help me track down the source of the problem. In cases where a person isn't swayed by the cultural current, studying their life patterns helps me identify what has kept them in the straight and narrow.

As I studied the lives of those in the Bible who fell from grace versus those who didn't, I realized the best defense against being swayed by the world came down to being comfortable in your own skin. The question then became, How do you develop internal strength that is not swayed by culture? To answer this question let's look at two Bible characters who faced intense pressure: one did not cave to the current of the world, and one did. This will reveal the determining factor that made a difference between the two.

EXAMPLE 1: KING HEZEKIAH

During his reign King Hezekiah faced a serious threat from Sennacherib, king of Assyria. With all eyes on him, King Hezekiah said,

> "Be strong and courageous. Do not be afraid or discouraged because of the king of Assyria and the vast army with him, for there is a greater power with us than with him. With him is only the arm of flesh, but with us is the LORD our God to help us and to fight our battles." And the people gained confidence from what Hezekiah the king of Judah said.
>
> —2 CHRONICLES 32:7–8

Later, the king of Assyria challenged Hezekiah's faith and tried to turn his own people against him. While under siege, Hezekiah kept the faith that regardless of his circumstances he served a God who had the capacity to deliver him. As things got worse, the Bible says,

> King Hezekiah and the prophet Isaiah son of Amoz cried out in prayer to heaven about this. And the LORD sent an angel, who annihilated all the fighting men and the commanders and officers in the camp of the Assyrian king. So he withdrew to his own land in disgrace. And when

he went into the temple of his god, some of his sons, his own flesh and blood, cut him down with the sword. So the LORD saved Hezekiah and the people of Jerusalem from the hand of Sennacherib king of Assyria and from the hand of all others. He took care of them on every side. Many brought offerings to Jerusalem for the LORD and valuable gifts for Hezekiah king of Judah. From then on he was highly regarded by all the nations.

—2 CHRONICLES 32:20–23

Hezekiah didn't take matters into his own hands, nor did he cave to the threats of man. Instead, he cried out to the One who could deliver him, believing that God would come through for him.

EXAMPLE 2: KING ASA

In the beginning Asa followed the Lord wholeheartedly. In fact, Scripture says,

Asa did what was good and right in the eyes of the LORD his God. He removed the foreign altars and the high places, smashed the sacred stones and cut down the Asherah poles. He commanded Judah to seek the LORD, the God of their ancestors, and to obey his laws and commands. He removed the high places and incense altars in every town in Judah, and the kingdom was at peace under him. He built up the fortified cities of Judah, since the land was at peace. No one was at war with him during those years, for the LORD gave him rest.

—2 CHRONICLES 14:2–6

When Asa faced a battle with Zerah the Cushite, the Bible says,

> Asa called to the LORD his God and said, "LORD, there is no one like you to help the powerless against the mighty. Help us, LORD our God, for we rely on you, and in your name we have come against this vast army. LORD, you are our God; do not let mere mortals prevail against you." The LORD struck down the Cushites before Asa and Judah. The Cushites fled....
>
> —2 CHRONICLES 14:11–12

Asa had a pattern of relying on the Lord, and the Lord giving him rest and victory, until all of a sudden—in the thirty-sixth year of his reign—as a response to an attack by an army,

> Asa then took the silver and gold out of the treasuries of the LORD's temple and of his own palace and sent it to Ben-Hadad king of Aram, who was ruling in Damascus. "Let there be a treaty between me and you," he said, "as there was between my father and your father. See, I am sending you silver and gold. Now break your treaty with Baasha king of Israel so he will withdraw from me."
>
> Ben-Hadad agreed with King Asa and sent the commanders of his forces against the towns of Israel. They conquered Ijon, Dan, Abel Maim and all the store cities of Naphtali. When Baasha heard this, he stopped building Ramah and abandoned

his work. Then King Asa brought all the men of Judah, and they carried away from Ramah the stones and timber Baasha had been using. With them he built up Geba and Mizpah.

At that time Hanani the seer came to Asa king of Judah and said to him: "Because you relied on the king of Aram and not on the LORD your God, the army of the king of Aram has escaped from your hand. Were not the Cushites and Libyans a mighty army with great numbers of chariots and horsemen? Yet when you relied on the LORD, he delivered them into your hand. For the eyes of the LORD range throughout the earth to strengthen those whose hearts are fully committed to him. You have done a foolish thing, and from now on you will be at war."

—2 CHRONICLES 16:2–9

Late in his reign Asa turned from relying on God to relying on people. After being confronted about his sin, instead of repenting, Asa put the messenger in prison. This led to his eventual illness and death.

As we see from these two people, true internal strength that allows a person to be comfortable with himself comes from a heart committed to God. I'm not talking about a mere verbal profession, because even Jesus said, "Many will say to me on that day, 'Lord, Lord, did we not prophesy in your name and in your name drive out demons and in your name perform many miracles?' Then I will tell them plainly, 'I never knew you. Away from me, you evildoers!'" (Matt. 7:22–24). I'm referring to a commitment to live for

Christ. That, my friend, is how we become comfortable in our own skin, not swayed by the current of the world.

DAVID: COMFORTABLE IN HIS OWN SKIN

David is a great example of someone who knew who he was in God. We see this specifically in the story of David and Goliath, when David was just a shepherd boy and he confronted a giant who threatened God's people. Before going up against Goliath, David sought permission from King Saul. David said to Saul,

> "Let no one lose heart on account of this Philistine; your servant will go and fight him." Saul replied, "You are not able to go out against this Philistine and fight him; you are only a young man, and he has been a warrior from his youth." But David said to Saul, "Your servant has been keeping his father's sheep. When a lion or a bear came and carried off a sheep from the flock, I went after it, struck it and rescued the sheep from its mouth. When it turned on me, I seized it by its hair, struck it and killed it. Your servant has killed both the lion and the bear; this uncircumcised Philistine will be like one of them, because he has defied the armies of the living God. The LORD who rescued me from the paw of the lion and the paw of the bear will rescue me from the hand of this Philistine."
>
> Saul said to David, "Go, and the LORD be with you." Then Saul dressed David in his own tunic. He put a coat of armor on him and a bronze

helmet on his head. David fastened on his sword over the tunic and tried walking around, because he was not used to them.

"I cannot go in these," he said to Saul, "because I am not used to them." So he took them off. Then he took his staff in his hand, chose five smooth stones from the stream, put them in the pouch of his shepherd's bag and, with his sling in his hand, approached the Philistine.

—1 SAMUEL 17:32–40

Just as God had placed certain gifts and skills to appropriate His calling on David's life, He did the same for you, and until you make a solid decision to live based on who God called you to be, you will risk trying to fit into everyone else's shoes and end up frustrated over and over when you don't. The truth is, the only shoes you're ever meant to fit into are the ones God called you to wear.

In studying people, I've found that those who try to live based on everyone else's expectations have greater chances of developing depression and anxiety-related disorders, because everyone has an opinion of who you should be and how you should act. In truth, the only One whose opinion of you and whose plans and purposes for you matter is the One who hung on the cross on your behalf. Jesus died and rose again so you might have the abundant life He purchased for you. But if you continue to live according to everyone else's expectations of you, you will miss out on living your life to its fullest.

Jesus said it this way: the devil comes to steal, kill, and destroy, but He came that you might have life and have it to the full (John 10:10). The prerequisite for experiencing fullness of life is that you be comfortable in your own skin. Being comfortable in your own skin requires you to know who you truly are in Jesus, which can only happen through a genuine and intimate relationship with your heavenly Father. David's confidence didn't come from thinking he was great but from knowing the greatness of the One he belonged to.

The Bible is very clear that David spent a lot of time with God. In fact, it seems from David's early life that he talked to God more than to anyone else. He sang songs to God expressing his complete trust in Him. Take a look at how he praises God in Psalm 145:14–19:

> The LORD upholds all who fall and lifts up all who are bowed down. The eyes of all look to you, and you give them their food at the proper time. You open your hand and satisfy the desires of every living thing. The LORD is righteous in all his ways and faithful in all he does. The LORD is near to all who call on him, to all who call on him in truth. He fulfills the desires of those who fear him; he hears their cry and saves them.

And in Psalm 146 (NLT) we read:

> Praise the LORD! Let all that I am praise the LORD. I will praise the LORD as long as I live. I will sing praises to my God with my dying breath. Don't put your confidence in powerful people; there is no help for you there. When they breathe their last, they return to the earth, and all their plans die with them. But joyful are those who have the

God of Israel as their helper, whose hope is in
the LORD their God. He made heaven and earth,
the sea, and everything in them. He keeps every
promise forever. He gives justice to the oppressed
and food to the hungry. The LORD frees the prisoners. The LORD opens the eyes of the blind. The
LORD lifts up those who are weighed down. The
LORD loves the godly. The LORD protects the for-
eigners among us. He cares for the orphans and
widows, but he frustrates the plans of the wicked.

David knew that if he was going to put hope in anyone,
it was the One who is worthy of it all—the Lord God
Almighty.

There were also times when David petitioned to God,
as we see in Psalm 143:8–10: "Let the morning bring me
word of your unfailing love, for I have put my trust in you.
Show me the way I should go, for to you I entrust my life.
Rescue me from my enemies, LORD, for I hide myself in
you. Teach me to do your will, for you are my God; may
your good Spirit lead me on level ground."

David had such a close, intimate relationship with God
that when faced with a threat, instead of looking at his
frailty, he looked to God's strength. In Psalm 144:1, David
speaks of the Lord this way: "Praise be to the LORD my
Rock, who trains my hands for war, my fingers for battle."
David was comfortable in his own skin because he knew
the One he belonged to and where his strength came from.

His interaction with Goliath reflected that:

[Goliath] looked David over and saw that he
was little more than a boy, glowing with health

and handsome, and he despised him. He said to David, "Am I a dog, that you come at me with sticks?" And the Philistine cursed David by his gods. "Come here," he said, "and I'll give your flesh to the birds and the wild animals!"

David said to the Philistine, "You come against me with sword and spear and javelin, but I come against you in the name of the LORD Almighty, the God of the armies of Israel, whom you have defied. This day the LORD will deliver you into my hands, and I'll strike you down and cut off your head. This very day I will give the carcasses of the Philistine army to the birds and the wild animals, and the whole world will know that there is a God in Israel. All those gathered here will know that it is not by sword or spear that the LORD saves; for the battle is the LORD's, and he will give all of you into our hands."

As the Philistine moved closer to attack him, David ran quickly toward the battle line to meet him. Reaching into his bag and taking out a stone, he slung it and struck the Philistine on the forehead. The stone sank into his forehead, and he fell facedown on the ground. So David triumphed over the Philistine with a sling and a stone; without a sword in his hand he struck down the Philistine and killed him.

—1 SAMUEL 17:42–50

This miraculous encounter goes to show that our inner strength is determined by how strong our confidence is in the Lord. The enemy wants you to build your inner strength on the foundation of people's praises so he can use those very people to bring you down. I once heard someone say if you live by people's praise you'll die by their criticism. The enemy knows the amount of influence people can have on our lives, especially if we're not grounded in God's love for us as our source of strength.

GROUNDED IN GOD'S STRENGTH

When David first looked into Goliath, his brothers made fun of him, treated him with contempt, and told him to go back to "those few sheep" he took care of (1 Sam. 17:28). Looking at this encounter, chances are this wasn't the first or last time David's brothers treated him this way. Had David's strength not been built on his confidence in the Lord and God's love for him, he would have caved at the sound of his brothers' criticism.

David's brothers weren't the only ones who didn't put much stock in him. Years earlier, when God sent the prophet Samuel to Jesse's house so He could show Samuel who he was to anoint as the next king, David's father (Jesse) didn't even bother to call David because he didn't consider him as an option for king.

> Jesse had seven of his sons pass before Samuel, but Samuel said to him, "The LORD has not chosen these." So he asked Jesse, "Are these all the sons you have?" "There is still the youngest," Jesse answered. "He is tending the sheep." Samuel said, "Send for him; we will not sit down until he arrives." So he sent for him and had him brought in. He was glowing with health and had a fine

appearance and handsome features. Then the
LORD said, "Rise and anoint him; this is the one."
—1 SAMUEL 16:10–12

How often does the enemy use situations where those
who are closest to you either attack you or weren't there
for you when you needed them, to try to convince you that
you'll never amount to anything. After all, "even those
who were supposed to love you can't find it in their hearts
to love you," he whispers in your ear, hoping you'll take
the bait and believe him. But know this: your heavenly
Father does not need anyone's permission to propel you
into everything He has planned for your life. No naysayers
and no powers of darkness can stop what God has in store
for you. Your part is to believe this to be true and to act
on this truth by putting your trust in Him, and Him alone.

QUESTIONS FOR REFLECTION

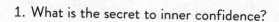

1. What is the secret to inner confidence?

2. What has kept you from developing inner confidence?

3. What steps do you plan to take moving forward to develop inner confidence?

Chapter 15

YOUR BATTLE PLAN AGAINST ENEMY 3

THERE IS A significant difference between loving people and putting our trust in them. Jesus loved people, but in John 2:24–25 we read, "Jesus would *not entrust himself to them*, for he knew all people. He did not need any testimony about mankind, for he knew what was in each person" (emphasis added). Loving people comes out of our relationship with God. "We love because he first loved us" (1 John 4:19). Putting our trust in people, however, comes out of a place of doubt in God. In our doubt, we create a plan B just in case God doesn't follow through on His promises. In our distrust, we look to people to fill shoes that only God can fill and set ourselves up to be disappointed.

Throughout my years as a therapist I've come to realize just how common it is for people to allow others to take God's spot in their lives, resulting in unnecessary mental torment. This led me to search for answers to questions such as, "What makes us want to put our trust in people rather than in God?" and "What makes us seek after God-substitutes to the point of compromising our relationship with God?"

After much prayer and research, the best I could find was (drumroll) our need for connection. You see, you and I were created for relationships. God intended for these healthy relationships to serve as a foundation for our connection with Him, leading us to develop a strong sense of identity. If you were brought up in a spiritually healthy environment, your parents likely modeled what a relationship with God looks like. They showed you grace when you needed it, held you accountable when you required it, disciplined you when you drifted away, modeled forgiveness to you when you messed up, and showed you mercy when you took a wrong turn.

Your understanding of the world is based on the frames of reference to which your brain has been exposed. If your upbringing looked like the example you just read, you were probably able to identify what a relationship with God looks like because you could use your parents as a frame of reference. It's much easier for someone to believe God is loving when a person in their lives has reflected God's love to them.

But if you experienced a series of traumatic events relating to those who were meant to protect you, out of sheer survival mechanism you will likely have difficulty trusting God. This doubt will either stem from fear of the unknown of what a relationship with God should look like, or it will stem from negative preconceived notions you hold about God. Since your yearning for connection doesn't go away, however, you will settle for fulfilling it through those around you, to no avail. This will lead to disappointment and—after rounds of disappointments—depression.

You may not be able to help how you were raised. As an adult, though, the responsibility rests on you to develop your own healthy relationship with God. I'm speaking to you from both personal and clinical experience. Your parents may not have given you a foundational frame of reference of what a healthy relationship with God looks like. But this doesn't mean you have to go the rest of your life without a healthy relationship with Him. James 4:8 says, "Come near to God and he will come near to you." God is knocking on the door of your heart right now. As Hebrews 3:15 says, "Today, if you hear his voice, do not harden your hearts."

God wants a relationship with you, a Father-child relationship. He is more than capable of satisfying every desire of your heart because He made you. When you do your part to seek after your heavenly Father, you will find that everything else in life, and everyone else in life, is just the cherry on top—a bonus from the Father. At the end of the day, He is the giver of everything good in our lives (Jas. 1:17).

In the last chapter we discussed the role inner confidence plays in defeating enemy 3. Now it's time to go over the practical steps needed to overcome this enemy. In other words, we're going to learn how to safeguard ourselves from becoming subject to external influence that would otherwise lead us astray.

1. Make time with God.

I emphasize *making* time for devotion because it's that important. Without intentionally setting aside time for God, you'll lose track of your day. You'll get to the end of your day and wonder where it went. At the risk of sounding harsh, you have to be willing to be real with yourself and ask if you're truly prioritizing God in your life—meaning, are you intentionally setting aside time to spend with Him not because you "have to" but because you "get to" do it?

Aside from the fact that we were made for God, the reason this is such an important step is because as we spend time with God we're able to learn about and experience His character. The closeness that develops overturns any negative frames of reference we previously held about Him. It also keeps us in a place of internal peace knowing that the King of kings—the powerful, faithful, almighty God who spoke worlds into existence—has our best interest at heart.

God needs to be number one in your life because He not only made you but also breathed the breath of life into you. David, whose inner confidence we used as an example in the previous chapter, once wrote, "For you created my inmost being; you knit me together in my mother's womb" (Ps. 139:13). He knows you inside and out. He knows everything about you. He knows you better than you'll ever know yourself. Jesus said, "Indeed, the very hairs of your head are all numbered. Don't be afraid; you are worth more than many sparrows" (Luke 12:7).

God is the One who made you for His plans and purposes. "For we are God's handiwork, created in Christ Jesus to do good works, which God prepared in advance for us to do" (Eph. 2:10). He is committed to seeing you through. As the apostle Paul wrote, "Being confident of this, that he who began a good work in you will carry it on to completion until the day of Christ Jesus" (Phil. 1:6). We usually get into trouble when we try to figure out our purpose before we ground ourselves in Christ. But "no one can lay any foundation other than the one already laid, which is Jesus Christ" (1 Cor. 3:11).

2. Define yourself by Him.

The world encourages you to define yourself by external factors. God is telling you to define yourself by Him.

As we saw in the Book of Ephesians, your identity precedes your behavior. Understanding who you are, and in particular whose you are, sets the tone for the kind of mindset you will hold throughout your life. When you surrendered your life to Jesus, God put His Holy Spirit within you, sealing you as His child. "When you believed, you were marked in him with a seal, the promised Holy Spirit, who is a deposit guaranteeing our inheritance until the redemption of those who are God's possession—to the praise of his glory" (Eph. 1:13–14).

Your relationship with God supersedes any earthly relationship you have. I genuinely believe the reason we elevate our earthly relationships to the point of idolizing them and compromising our relationship with God is because we don't understand the love God extends to us through Christ. Although we are born again, we continue to live as sheep without a shepherd. And because we were made for a Shepherd, we end up looking to those around us to fulfill what only God can.

3. Pray Ephesians 3:14–21.

When Satan tempted Jesus, Jesus answered him with "It is written...." One of the greatest passages to use to combat the devil is Ephesians 3:14–21. I encourage you to pray this powerful prayer over your life every day (eventually you will memorize it). This Scripture passage will not only remind you of God's love for you; but when the enemy tries to entice you or make you seek security in people, it will be in your heart. It will shield you from allowing people's influence to surpass God's influence. Let's look at it now:

> For this reason I kneel before the Father, from whom every family in heaven and on earth derives its name. I pray that out of his glorious riches he may strengthen you with power through his Spirit in your inner being, so that Christ may dwell in your hearts through faith. And I pray that you, being rooted and established in love, may have power, together with all the Lord's holy people, to grasp how wide and long and high and deep is the love of Christ, and to know this love that surpasses knowledge—that you may be filled to the measure of all the fullness of God.
>
> Now to him who is able to do immeasurably more than all we ask or imagine, according to his power that is at work within us, to him be glory in the church and in Christ Jesus throughout all generations, for ever and ever! Amen.

David once said it this way: "I have hidden your word in my heart that I might not sin against you" (Ps. 119:11).

4. Identify "That person/Those people."

Continuing with self-reflection, I have listed several indicators to help you discern whether someone has taken God's place in your life (intentionally or unintentionally). Please note: it's helpful to replace the words "that person" with the person's name or the object's name.

- I look to *that person* for direction in my life.

- I ask myself, "How would *that person* feel about me doing this?"

- I've changed my opinion about something because *that person* didn't agree with my previous opinion.

- When *that person* is upset with me, I have a hard time resting until our relationship is OK, regardless of whether their anger toward me was my fault or not.

- *That person* can affect my mood throughout the day.

- I talk to *that person* more than I talk to God.

If you believe you've fallen into the trap of putting people in your God spot, your next step is to renounce idolatry of man from your heart by praying the following prayer.

Father God, I come to You with a humble heart, knowing that my actions have broken Your heart. Lord, forgive me for my many sins. I declare that You are the King of kings and Lord of lords, the Alpha and Omega, the beginning and the end. There's nothing that is too hard for You. Lord, forgive me for elevating man to a place where only You belong. Right now by Your Holy Spirit, please search my heart and reveal to me anyone I have put on a pedestal in my heart. (Wait for God to show you. When He does, continue.) Father, forgive me for putting (name) on a pedestal, for You alone are worthy of my praise, You alone are worthy of my worship, You alone are worthy of my faith.

In the coming days, weeks, and months, please show me how (name)'s opinions have affected me in the way I think and the path I'm taking. Lord, I desire nothing more than You. Like David, teach me to do Your will, for You are the God of my salvation, and on You I wait all day. Lord God, lead me by Your truth and teach me. Teach me how to rely on the Holy Spirit and how to have fellowship with You and the Holy Spirit. Teach me how to wait on the Holy Spirit to hear His promptings. My relationship with You is my everything. Teach me how to grow in my relationship with You. In times when I mess up, help me remember that You convict me because You love me. And when the enemy tries to sweep in with words of condemnation, I pray that You will silence his voice and bring to mind Your truth in my heart—that You, my Father, who began a good work in me, are faithful to complete it until either You call me home with You in glory or Jesus comes back. Amen.

PART IV
WEAPONS OF WARFARE

Chapter 16

THERE'S A TARGET
ON YOUR BACK

AS A COUNSELOR, one of the most frequent questions I hear regarding spiritual attacks on the mind is "When does it get better?" Unfortunately, while we live on this side of eternity, the enemy will always have a target on our backs. But Jesus said in Him we have power to trample lions and scorpions (Luke 10:19). In other words, the enemy is never going to stop attacking us, but in Christ we're never defenseless. Now that we've gone through each one of the three enemies and how to defeat them when they arise, I'd like to give you a few principles to keep at the forefront of your mind when the enemy comes knocking, because he will.

1. Leave no room for the enemy to try to wiggle his way into your life. Surrender every aspect of your life to God and ask Him to reorganize it according to how He wants it to be.

This is one of the scariest petitions you can make of God because you're essentially asking the Holy Spirit to take an inventory of your life and prune what needs to be pruned. Why? So that you might live a life worthy of the call God has put on it.

This inventory includes every role you currently occupy, starting with the most important role: His child. If you are married, it includes your role as a spouse. If you have children, it includes your role as a parent. It also includes your roles as friend, coworker, and so forth. We're often afraid to ask God to take inventory of our lives and do with us as He wishes because we're scared He's going to wreak havoc on our lives. That's not who God is.

Surrendering every aspect of your life reminds the devil, your flesh, and everyone else around you ("the world") that the Lord Jesus Christ is your God—and that your life belongs to Him and Him alone.

The Word says that life is fleeting. How often do we waste precious time God has allotted us worrying about the wrong things or focusing on the wrong stuff?

Years ago I developed pain in my leg. The pain started as a dull ache in my lower back. As time went on, however, it got worse and radiated down my leg, causing sharp shooting pains. I decided to confide in my friend about it, as she had experienced something similar years before. My friend suggested seeing a chiropractor because she had experienced good results herself.

Taking her advice, I wasted no time in making an appointment with a chiropractor. During my visit the doctor examined my back and decided to take an X-ray to get a better understanding of the underlying issue. To my surprise, the X-ray revealed that my spine was misaligned, causing a nerve to be pinched and resulting in the shooting pains down my leg.

With the diagnosis in hand, the chiropractor started treatment. Through a series of adjustments, he realigned my spine, relieving the pressure on the affected nerve. At first I experienced soreness after the adjustments since my nerves were used to being out of alignment. But with each treatment they gradually settled into their correct positions.

After a few sessions the pain that had plagued me for so long stopped. The chiropractor also gave me exercises and stretches to strengthen my back and prevent any future issues.

Surrendering every aspect of our lives to God works in a similar way. Anything out of alignment with His will causes problems. Just like my pain, this process usually starts small until we stray from God's will in one area. As a result, other areas of our lives feel pressure. That's why it's so important to make a habit of asking God to examine every area of our lives.

Will inviting God to realign our lives be a quick adjustment? I don't know. But here's what I can tell you: your Father, the God who brought the world into existence, loves you more than anyone ever could. And regardless of how off-track your life may be, when you ask Him to realign it, you can rest assured that you're entrusting it into the safest, most caring, most trustworthy, and most capable hands imaginable.

If you'd like to ask God to realign your life according to how He sees fit, pray this prayer:

> *Faithful Father, You are mighty and sovereign. You are all-wise and all-knowing. I surrender into Your hands every aspect of my life and declare that my mind is Yours, my heart is Yours, and every part of me is Yours. Lord, I confess that throughout my life I've done*

things I shouldn't have, said things I shouldn't have, and thought things I shouldn't have. Yet through it all You've been faithful to look out for me. Father, You are worthy of every aspect of my life. Forgive me for using my time in ways that have not honored You. Forgive me for being distracted by things that are meaningless, and forgive me for all the times I've gotten carried away with meaningless conversations, gossip, slander, and anything that did not honor You.

Holy Spirit, renew my mind. More than anything, I want to have the mind of Christ. I want people to look at me and know that I am Yours by word and deed, so please give me eyes that are focused on You and You alone. When distraction comes my way, Father, strengthen me to keep my eyes on You, the author and finisher of my faith. Give me singleness of heart so that I elevate Your will over my own will and over people's expectations for my life.

Lord, when You lead me to have difficult conversations or to say no to something, strengthen me and give me boldness to speak Your truth in love. When the enemy whispers thoughts of guilt for standing my ground, remind me of Your truth. Help me remember that it's OK to say no to things that may seem good but aren't part of Your plan for me. Father, in the mighty name of Jesus, I invite You into my friendships. Prune away people in my life who are leading me astray from You, and bring forth friendships that will help me grow in You.

Lord, whenever I fall and You convict me, I pray that I will be quick to repent and see Your love in Your discipline. Strengthen my hands for battle and help me to use the weapons of warfare You have equipped me with to ward off the attacks of the enemy. I pray that You will give me wisdom beyond my years to fill every role You have called me to fill.

Lord, please put Your desires for my life in my heart. Give me a hunger for Your Word and close my appetite to what the world has to offer.

Teach me to do Your will. Help me and strengthen me to stay on the path You've laid out for me. I pray that my actions would be pleasing to You. I pray that my legacy would be one of a man/woman after the Father's heart. Most of all, when You call me home, I pray that I will hear You say, "Well done, good and faithful servant." I pray this in the mighty name of Jesus. Amen.

2. Make praise a part of your everyday vocabulary. The enemy doesn't have any new tricks, so you want to pay attention to where he attacks you most. For example, he likes to sneak up on me with anxiety, especially when I have a lot going on that is not within my control. One time when I was preparing a piece on spiritual warfare, the enemy would not let up. He bombarded me with flashbacks of traumatic situations in my life that I hadn't even thought about for years—things I had forgiven and long forgotten. He put horrible images in my mind of what-if scenarios, all the awful things that could ever go wrong.

And of course he came at me with this at night. Don't you love it when he does that? You're already exhausted and trying to sleep. You have an early morning ahead. So he decides to bug you and steal your rest.

That night I prayed that the Lord would set up a wall of fire around my home and send mighty angels to encamp at every corner of my house. I pleaded the blood of Jesus over my home and anointed my whole house. The next morning the Lord woke me up at 4 a.m. and led me to a passage in 2 Chronicles 20. The passage recalls a time when the people of Judah, under the reign of King Jehoshaphat, were being attacked by a coalition of enemies. In that passage the Lord spoke to a prophet and told him to reassure the king and the people. In verses 15–17 the prophet said:

> Listen, King Jehoshaphat and all who live in Judah and Jerusalem! This is what the LORD says to you: "Do not be afraid or discouraged because of this vast army. For the battle is not yours, but God's. Tomorrow march down against them. They will be climbing up by the Pass of Ziz, and you will find them at the end of the gorge in the Desert of Jeruel. You will not have to fight this battle. Take up your positions; stand firm and see the deliverance the LORD will give you, Judah and Jerusalem. Do not be afraid; do not be discouraged. Go out to face them tomorrow, and the LORD will be with you."

Verses 18–19 show that in response to the Lord's assurance, "Jehoshaphat bowed down with his face to the ground, and all the people of Judah and Jerusalem fell down in worship before the LORD. Then some Levites from the Kohathites and Korahites stood up and praised the LORD, the God of Israel, with a very loud voice."

The story continues in verses 20–22:

> As they set out, Jehoshaphat stood and said, "Listen to me, Judah and people of Jerusalem! Have faith in the LORD your God and you will be upheld; have faith in his prophets and you will be successful." After consulting the people, Jehoshaphat appointed men to sing to the LORD and to praise him for the splendor of his holiness as they went out at the head of the army, saying: "Give thanks to the LORD, for his love endures forever." As they began to sing and praise, the LORD set ambushes against the men of Ammon and Moab and Mount Seir who were invading Judah, and they were defeated.

That morning the Lord showed me how so often when we get attacked one of the first things that goes out the window is our faith. We forget whom we belong to and crumble in fear—exactly what the enemy wants us to do! Instead, we are to do what Jehoshaphat and the people of Judah and Jerusalem did: praise Him. He reassures us that He is with us. Our job is to spend time with Him and believe Him. And if we have trouble believing Him, something I've found helpful in the midst of trial is to write down the last three times the Lord brought me through something really hard. Remembering God's faithfulness will help your faith, because even when we are faithless, He remains faithful (2 Tim. 2:13).

The second thing the Lord highlighted to me in this passage is that praise is the grenade that tears the enemy's camp to shreds. The Bible says that God inhabits the praises of His people (Ps. 22:3). When you start praising God, regardless of your circumstances, you're proclaiming God's glory and presence over whatever chaos the enemy is trying to create. When you praise the name of Jesus, the devil and his angels have two choices: either to kneel or to flee.

The third thing the Lord showed me is the actual words of praise the people of Judah and Jerusalem were speaking. Not only did they exalt the name of the Lord, but they affirmed that, regardless of their circumstances, God's love endured. That means no matter what my situation looks like, I know my Redeemer lives. No matter what is going on, "I am convinced that neither death nor life, neither angels nor demons, neither the present nor the future, nor any powers, neither height nor depth, nor anything else in all creation, will be able to separate us from the love of God that is in Christ Jesus our Lord" (Rom. 8:38–39).

I'm sharing this with you because on this side of eternity the enemy will keep coming after us, and sometimes God will allow us to walk through hard seasons; but as you're walking through them you have to strengthen yourself in the Lord. Remind yourself that God has not given you a spirit of bondage again to fear. He's given you a spirit of adoption by whom you cry out, "Abba, Father" (Rom. 8:15).

Remind yourself that, regardless of your circumstances, you have a Father to whom you belong. A Father who chose you to be His before the foundation of the world. A Father who watched over you as He knit you together in your mother's womb. A Father who pursued you even when you wanted nothing to do with Him.

YOUR FATHER IS CALLING

A few years before I surrendered my life to Jesus, the Lord gave me a series of recurring dreams. All of them had the same theme. I already shared the one about receiving a letter from a king. Another dream went like this: I would be asleep and hear the phone ringing loudly, and someone would answer it, saying, "Kenza, your Father is calling you." I had that dream at least four or five times in a row. Because the enemy had a veil over my eyes, I didn't catch on to what the dream meant. Years later I realized that my Father in heaven was calling me to Him before I came to know Him.

The same goes for you. Your heavenly Father has never stopped pursuing you. If you look back on your life, you'll realize how He orchestrated certain events and placed certain people in your path to point you to Him. Your Father moved heaven and earth to have a relationship with you, so don't let a worthless demon convince you otherwise.

The devil loves to come in the midst of the chaos he created to try to get you to believe lies such as "God must have left you" or "If God cared about you, why would He allow such and such to happen?" or "Where is your God now?"

It is during these times that you must stand on your own two feet and praise the Father. Say, "Father, I praise You. Lord Jesus, I declare that You are the King of kings and Lord of lords. I thank You that You are the Alpha and Omega and that You hold the beginning and the end.

Thank You that You are all-powerful and greater than all the powers of darkness combined. Thank You, Lord, that no one can compare with You. Thank You that nothing can separate me from Your love in Christ Jesus. Thank You that Your Word never returns void. Thank You, Lord, that Your love for me is incomprehensible. Thank You that Your presence brings me unspeakable joy. Thank You, Lord Jesus, that through Your death and resurrection I have been set free from the powers of darkness and that no weapon formed against me will prosper.

"Thank You that in You I live and move and have my being. Thank You, Father God, that when I sleep You are with me; when I wake up You are with me; and You never cease to look out for me. Thank You for loving me and rescuing me. Lord Jesus, You are worthy. King Jesus, I am forever indebted to You. Lord Jesus, I praise You. My heart is Yours. My mind is Yours. All that I am is Yours. To You be the praise and honor and glory forever and ever. Amen!"

3. Surround yourself with a healthy community of believers (with the expectation that they are not perfect). The goal of fellowship and unity with brothers and sisters in Christ is for them to support our relationship with God, not be a substitute for it. If we don't take the time to get to know God's character and learn to draw strength from Him, we will risk putting people in our God spot again and going back to the destructive cycle of the world. God puts people in our lives at various times for distinct reasons. The following are the two most common reasons God may put someone in your life.

Encouragement

God is our source of strength. At times He uses people to help encourage us when we're down. God may use people as vessels to speak truth into our lives and remind us of who we are in Him when we have forgotten. A few years ago I was asked to speak at an interfaith conference. I was so excited about the opportunity, mainly because I was going to share about my two favorite topics: God and mental health.

The week leading up to the conference, the devil caused chaos in multiple areas of my life. My husband and I stayed up all night praying, and by that morning I was physically and emotionally drained. I was scheduled to deliver a message I felt God had put on my heart for that day, and as my husband prayed over me, God brought a friend to mind. This friend is a prayer warrior, so I called her and told her what was going on. My friend reminded me of my place in Christ versus the enemy's place. The way she encouraged me that morning could have only come from the throne room of heaven. I believe God used her as a conduit of encouragement to me. She said the right things for me to be able to jump out of bed, get dressed, show up at the conference, and deliver the word God had put on my heart for the people that day.

The whole time I prepared for the conference, I thought I was going to be one of many speakers bringing the Word. It wasn't until I got there that I realized this conference hosted people of many faiths. This, of course, didn't change my speech; what it did was stir up my faith. I finally realized why the enemy had attacked me all night and created chaos in my life for most of the week. Thinking that I was going to be speaking to and encouraging people in the faith, I let my guard down, which we're never to do. My whole speech was about the powerful love of God. Little did I know I was speaking to people who saw God as harsh—a dictator—and people who didn't believe in Him at all. Though I didn't know this, God did and prepared the way, and though the enemy harassed me all night, God led my husband to pray over me without ceasing that night, and He provided my friend's encouragement to launch me into the conference.

Looking back, were my husband and my friend the sources of encouragement? To the naked eye they may have been. But in reality they were conduits of God's encouragement to me that day. God knows exactly what you need to hear and when you need to hear it, and at times He will use people to deliver His message. At the end of the day He remains the true source.

Accountability

God can also use people to hold us accountable. That's where life groups or Bible study groups come in. Not only do they serve as a resource for equipping us with God's Word, but they hold us accountable to the call of God on our lives.

Remember: the people in our Bible study groups will not be perfect. Now that doesn't mean that if your Bible study group likes to go out drinking it's the right group for you! That's where your relationship with God comes in. He will give you the discernment you need to choose the right group for your current season of life.

Throughout the years my husband and I have been in several different Bible study groups. When we first got married most of our group consisted of single or newly married people. When we started having children, we slowly transitioned into a group with parents who had children the same age as ours or older. Transitions like these can often bring about some distress, because as human beings we don't like change.

If this is where you find yourself in life, just remember to give yourself grace. And remind yourself that if God is calling you out of one group into another, it doesn't mean you're no longer friends with the first group. It just means you've entered into a new season of equipping, and the new group will serve you better now.

Regardless of which community group we are connected to during any season of life, God is our ultimate anchor. Jesus is the vine, and we are the branches (John 15:5). Keep in mind that no matter how great someone may seem they must never take God's place in your life. God is your source. Everyone else, including you, is a resource God uses to bring the body together to carry out His plans and purposes until He either calls us home or Jesus comes back. The ultimate goal of our relationships is to draw one another toward a closer relationship with God, who called us out of darkness into His marvelous light.

WHEN IS IT TIME TO SEEK HELP?

Before I close out this book, I'd like to note that on some occasions we may experience depression that is clinical in nature. When we ask God to search our hearts, we find that the depression has nothing to do with our misstep with God but is the result of living in a broken world. The Bible recounts the stories of many individuals who suffered clinical depression as a direct result of grief or persecution for their faith.

One example that stands out is Job. The Bible makes it clear that Job's depression had nothing to do with disobeying God but was a direct result of the loss he experienced in his life. Another example is the prophet Jeremiah. He experienced depression to the point of becoming suicidal, not because he disobeyed God, but because he was being persecuted for his faith.

These examples show that clinical depression is not always the result of our not walking with God. Sometimes God allows difficult circumstances in our lives. During these hardships it's so important that we are grounded in Him so our hardships do not sway us. And when we experience hardships, our friends (like Job's friends) may look down on us and attribute our depression to being out of alignment with God.

This is why it's so important that we are rooted and grounded in God's love. When trials and tribulations come, we can confidently stand on Romans 8:28: "And we know that in all things God works for the good of those who love him, who have been called according to his purpose."

In other words, if your Father has allowed it in your life, He will bring you through it, and you can be sure something good will come from it. You may not see the good now or know about it on this side of eternity, but rest assured that God is faithful to His Word. Something good will come out of your pain.

FINAL EXHORTATION

W<small>E OFTEN BELIEVE</small> that once we give our lives to Jesus we don't have to struggle with the three enemies we discussed in this book. The reality is just the opposite. When we belong to Christ, though Satan knows he can't take us out, he will try to sway us to put our faith in things God considers an abomination, things we went over in part 1. If he can't convince us to do that, he will try to persuade us to put too much confidence in ourselves to lead us into destruction, because he knows we are no match for him. If he can't convince us to do that, he will draw on the power of relationships by using people to pull us away from our relationship with God.

Long before Satan attempted to use the three-enemies tactic with us, God outlined it in Jeremiah 17:5–8. Take a look below:

> This is what the L<small>ORD</small> says: "Cursed is the one who trusts in man, who draws strength from mere flesh and whose heart turns away from the L<small>ORD</small>. That person will be like a bush in the wastelands; they will not see prosperity when it comes. They will dwell in the parched places of the desert, in a salt land where no one lives.
>
> "But blessed is the one who trusts in the L<small>ORD</small>, whose confidence is in him. They will be like a

tree planted by the water that sends out its roots by the stream. It does not fear when heat comes; its leaves are always green. It has no worries in a year of drought and never fails to bear fruit."

As you see from this passage, the best weapon of defense against the enemy is our faith in Jesus. We must continuously fill our hearts with God's Word and remain in His love. We need to stay in tune with His voice every single day of our lives. God promises He will never leave us or forsake us, and He is true to His Word. It's time we do our part and stand on it.

I pray that this book has spurred your spirit to draw near to the One who calls you by name. May you walk with Him all the days of your life and remain aware of His everlasting love for you. In Jesus' name, amen.

NOTES

CHAPTER 6

1. "1 Samuel 10," *Matthew Henry's Commentary on the Whole Bible*, Bible Study Tools, accessed February 22, 2024, https://www.biblestudytools.com/commentaries/matthew-henry-concise/1-samuel/10.html.

CHAPTER 11

1. "Major Depression," National Institute of Mental Health, accessed January 25, 2024, https://www.nimh.nih.gov/health/statistics/major-depression.

CHAPTER 13

1. See Gary Chapman, *The 5 Love Languages: The Secret to Love That Lasts* (Northfield Publishing, 2010).

ABOUT THE AUTHOR

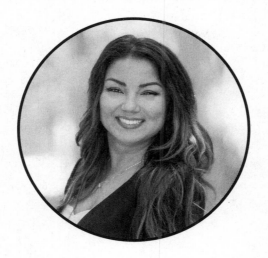

Kenza Haddock, LPCS, BCPC, is a licensed professional counselor and an accredited clinical trauma specialist with expertise in treating complex mental health conditions through both clinical and biblical methods. A former Muslim, she has spoken at conferences and churches and has been featured in numerous news outlets regarding the intersection of Christianity and mental health counseling. Kenza and her husband own Oceanic Counseling Group LLC, an outpatient mental health agency headquartered in South Carolina.

Kenza is passionate about empowering her readers with practical strategies to navigate and overcome a range of mental health challenges in their day-to-day lives. To learn more about her work or to connect with Kenza, visit her on Facebook at www.facebook.com/kenzahaddock or go to her website at www.kenzahaddock.com.